Praise for **Living Well**

"Dr. Abramowitz has the best grasp of O
who doesn't have OCD themselves. He a
people skirt around. This makes a world ⟨
trust him. Dr. Abramowitz provides validation and tangible guidance to
navigate times when OCD makes 'normal' hard life events even harder."
             —Callie C., Winston-Salem, North Carolina

"If you want an artfully written guide to OCD that's still research based,
this is the book for you. Dr. Abramowitz provides skills to help you push
back against OCD and live the life you want. Family members will find
insight, too. A 'must read!'"
             —Eric A. Storch, PhD, McIngvale Presidential
                 Endowed Chair and Professor of Psychiatry,
                 Baylor College of Medicine

"Getting effective treatment for OCD can substantially reduce your
symptoms, but there is more to life than that—like developing healthy
relationships, pursuing joy and meaning, and practicing self-compassion.
Living Well with OCD covers all of this and a whole lot more! This
research-based book is one-stop shopping for anyone with OCD."
             —C. Alec Pollard, PhD, Founding Director,
                 Center for OCD and Anxiety-Related Disorders,
                 Saint Louis Behavioral Medicine Institute

"Dr. Abramowitz knows that even if you've benefited from evidence-
based treatment for OCD, you need additional strategies to deal with
both everyday stresses and bigger life changes. This book gives you a
clear understanding and a step-by-step approach for addressing any OCD
triggers that come up, even unexpected ones. I couldn't recommend this
book more!"
             —Elizabeth McIngvale, PhD, LCSW, Director,
                 OCD Institute of Texas

"An indispensable resource for anyone grappling with the persistent daily
impact of OCD. Whether you're currently in treatment or seeking additional support, this guide is invaluable for achieving a more balanced,
fulfilling existence. I strongly recommend it."
             —Jenny Yip, PsyD, ABPP, author of *Hello Baby,
                 Goodbye Intrusive Thoughts*

THE GUILFORD LIVING WELL SERIES

The Guilford Living Well Series is designed to help individuals with common psychological conditions solve everyday problems and optimize their quality of life. Readers get specific, empathic advice for stress-proofing daily routines; navigating work, family, and relationship issues; managing symptoms effectively; and finding answers to treatment questions. Written by leading experts on each disorder, books in the series are concise, practical, and empowering.

Living Well with Bipolar Disorder
David J. Miklowitz

Living Well with OCD
Jonathan S. Abramowitz

FORTHCOMING

Living Well with Social Anxiety
Deborah Dobson

Living Well with ADHD
Laura E. Knouse

Living Well with Psychosis
Aaron P. Brinen

Living Well with Depression
Christopher R. Martell

living well with OCD

Also from Jonathan S. Abramowitz

FOR GENERAL READERS

Getting Over OCD: A 10-Step Workbook for Taking Back
Your Life, Second Edition

The Family Guide to Getting Over OCD:
Reclaim Your Life and Help Your Loved One

The Stress Less Workbook: Simple Strategies to Relieve
Pressure, Manage Commitments, and Minimize Conflicts

FOR PROFESSIONALS

Exposure Therapy for Anxiety:
Principles and Practice, Second Edition
Jonathan S. Abramowitz, Brett J. Deacon,
and Stephen P. H. Whiteside

living well *with*

OCD

PRACTICAL STRATEGIES FOR IMPROVING YOUR DAILY LIFE

JONATHAN S. ABRAMOWITZ, PhD

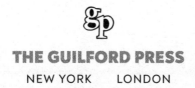

THE GUILFORD PRESS

NEW YORK   LONDON

Copyright © 2025 The Guilford Press
A Division of Guilford Publications, Inc.
www.guilford.com

Library of Congress Cataloging-in-Publication Data is available from the publisher.

ISBN 978-1-4625-5376-1 (paperback) — ISBN 978-1-4625-5654-0 (hardcover)

Author's note: The illustrations and examples in this book are thoroughly disguised
to protect individuals' privacy or are composites of real people.

contents

Introduction   1

1   Charting a path to living well   7

2   Replacing shame and guilt with self-compassion   21

3   Quieting obsessional fears and doubts   36

4   Riding out compulsive urges   51

5   Taking control of your time   67

6   Finding a balance between privacy and disclosure   83

7   Getting the healthy support you deserve   99

8   Maintaining family harmony   115

9   Thriving in romantic relationships   130

10 Navigating work and school   149

11 Surviving a crisis   164

12 Rethinking treatment   179

Index   199

About the author   208

Purchasers of this book can download and print select materials at *www.guilford.com/abramowitz5-forms* for personal use or use with clients (see copyright page for details).

introduction

Pick up any book or scientific article about obsessive–compulsive disorder (OCD) and you'll see statistics showing that this disorder is among the most common and disabling mental health conditions, affecting 2–3% of the population (that's over one million people in the United States) and costing the health care system loads of money. You'll read how OCD is a lifelong problem that interferes not only with work and school, but also with social activities and personal relationships. You'll also learn that OCD is associated with increased rates of anxiety, depression, and even suicide, and that we need more research to develop new and more effective treatments. There's no doubt that all of this information is true, and yet there are virtually no books or research articles that address the question most vital to the scores of people living with this disorder: *How can I lead a better life despite having OCD?*

The good news is that OCD is no longer the "lifetime sentence" it once was. For decades, it was "treated" using unscientific Freudian psychoanalysis, which simply wasn't effective. In the 1960s, however, scientific psychologists developed exposure and response prevention (ERP), a type of cognitive-behavioral therapy (CBT) that research has shown to be very helpful for OCD. In the 1970s and 1980s, studies showed that selective serotonin reuptake inhibitors (SSRIs) could also help reduce OCD symptoms. But neither ERP nor SSRIs are perfect solutions by any stretch. The SSRIs often produce annoying side effects, and ERP requires that you repeatedly face the situations and thoughts that trigger obsessional fears (exposure) while resisting the urge to perform compulsive rituals (response prevention)—not exactly a walk in the park! Moreover, while these treatments directly target OCD symptoms, they aren't broad enough to address all the problems with daily living and other important areas of life that OCD often disrupts, such as your self-esteem and your ability to maintain satisfying relationships. Finally, the fact is that these treatments don't work for everyone; and when they do work, they often have only partial effects. As a result, there are many more people living with OCD than those who have overcome it—and that's why I've written this book.

Let me be perfectly clear: If you've been diagnosed with OCD, I strongly recommend considering ERP or medication first. They are the most thoroughly researched treatments and the ones most likely to bring you relief. *Period.* Yet ERP is hard work, and properly carrying it out—with a therapist or with a self-help book—can be challenging. I don't blame anyone who feels they simply aren't ready to face their fears while giving up their rituals. Fortunately, there are second-line psychotherapies and biological approaches that may be worth trying if that's the case. But even if you've responded well to any treatment, there will still be lingering effects from having OCD that you'll need other tools and strategies to address, because these effects fall beyond the reach of therapies that target OCD itself. The aim of this book is to give you those tools and strategies as solutions to specific problems that keep you from living well. Thus you can use this book as a resource whether or not you've received treatment.

Do you feel wiped out from wrestling with lingering obsessional thoughts and doubts? Do you struggle to do things on time because of compulsive rituals or avoidance strategies? Maybe obsessions and rituals make family relationships awkward or perhaps interfere with your romantic life, intimacy, and sex. Does OCD make it difficult to navigate work or school or to manage when an unexpected crisis hits? Lots of people with this disorder get down on themselves—do you often feel shame and guilt? Wouldn't it be nice to have a strong network of people you can trust and turn to for support? This book contains strategies and exercises for solving these (and other) problems so you can achieve a better quality of life despite your OCD symptoms. As mentioned, these strategies and exercises are separate from ERP but can be helpful even if you haven't received that treatment. And if you *have* tried ERP or medications (or any other therapies), they'll complement these treatments to help you achieve more complete and enduring results.

Who Am I?

This seems like a good spot to introduce myself and tell you about my work in the field of OCD. My journey began in the 1990s when, as a student, I had remarkable opportunities to learn about OCD by working on research studies, providing lots of therapy, and receiving close mentorship and supervision from some of the world's leading experts on this disorder, including Drs. Edna Foa, Michael Kozak, and Martin Franklin. In 2000 I opened my own OCD research and treatment program at the Mayo Clinic and personally consulted with and treated hundreds of patients, while training and supervising many students and professionals. I also published my first three books on OCD while at Mayo, putting what I had learned though my research, training, and clinical work into print so others could benefit.

In 2006 I moved my clinic and research team to the University of North Carolina at Chapel Hill, where I am a professor and serve as director of the clinical psychology PhD program. I am passionate about training and supervising the "OCD experts of tomorrow," learning new information through research, and teaching clinicians how to implement effective treatment. I also have a small practice that I devote almost exclusively to treating people with OCD who come to Chapel Hill from across the region for my services.

Throughout my career, I have learned so much about OCD from my patients. In fact, they have been my best teachers. By paying close attention to their experiences, I have gained invaluable insights into OCD. This patient-centered approach has allowed me to use my clinical skills and research knowledge to help them more effectively. Understanding their unique experiences has been essential in developing and refining treatment strategies that truly address their needs.

You may be familiar with my other books on OCD: *Getting Over OCD: A 10-Step Workbook for Taking Back Your Life* (2nd edition, Guilford Press, 2019) and *The Family Guide to Getting Over OCD: Reclaim Your Life and Help Your Loved One* (Guilford Press, 2021). *Getting Over OCD* is a workbook that walks readers through an ERP-based self-help treatment program. *The Family Guide to Getting Over OCD* offers information and advice for readers who live with a loved one with OCD. But knowing that so many people are living with OCD symptoms I felt it was important to write a book that provides focused solutions for the day-to-day problems that this disorder creates.

What's in This Book?

The chapters in this book provide you with strategies you'll use to manage the ongoing complications that often arise as a result of having OCD. You'll probably find yourself trying different strategies until you land on the ones that help you the most. To ensure that you get the most out of them, each chapter ends with "Practical Steps to Living Well," a list of tips for making your efforts as successful as possible. You can download and print them to post somewhere you'll see them or to carry with you as reminders (see *www.guilford.com/abramowitz5-forms*).

You'll begin your journey toward living well with OCD by learning about what's required to overcome this disorder and why its symptoms might continue to create problems whether or not you have received treatment (Chapter 1). Chapter 2 helps you cultivate resilience and self-acceptance to combat feelings of guilt, shame, and self-stigma that often go along with OCD. From there you'll learn various skills—other than those acquired in ERP—that you can use when stubborn obsessional thinking and compulsive urges pop up and begin competing for your time (Chapters 3, 4, and 5).

OCD affects social relationships in numerous ways, which is why four chapters are dedicated to navigating specific interpersonal challenges. Chapter 6 offers suggestions for whether, when, and how to tactfully discuss your OCD symptoms with others. In Chapter 7, you'll learn about healthy support networks and how you can get help and inspiration through beneficial connections with peers, professionals, groups, and organizations. OCD also affects family relationships. In Chapter 8 you'll find strategies for communicating in healthy ways and reducing family conflict so you and your family can work together to help you (and them) live well. Finally, OCD can be a third wheel in your romantic relationship, so in Chapter 9 I offer tools for keeping OCD from interfering with areas of life such as dating, intimacy, and sex.

If you're in school, you might be able to get accommodations so that OCD doesn't stop you from performing at your full potential. And did you know there are laws that pertain to the rights of people with mental disorders in the workplace? Chapter 10 offers suggestions for how to make sure OCD doesn't derail your academic or work productivity. Chapter 11 helps you manage crisis situations when you're feeling overwhelmed with anxiety. There I provide practical suggestions you can use in the heat of any moment. The final chapter of the book, Chapter 12, focuses on strategies that help you optimize the effects of treatment if you are currently receiving ERP or medication. And if you haven't been inclined to try ERP or SSRIs before, or you're on the fence about returning to these treatments because you feel you didn't get much out of them, perhaps by the time you've gone through this book you'll find yourself reconsidering.

Even if that's not the case right now, the strategies in the following chapters can help you improve your quality of life. Please remember that you are not defined by your OCD, but by the strength, resilience, and determination you demonstrate on your journey toward a life filled with ambitions and accomplishments.

1

charting a path to living well

Your journey toward living well despite having OCD begins with understanding how this disorder forms a vicious cycle that leads to difficulties in your day-to-day life. Even if you've received treatment, lingering symptoms and ripple effects may pop up in your workday, at home with your family, in your relationships with friends and romantic partners, and in your attempts to enjoy leisure time and tend to your personal well-being. Having insight into how this happens is the foundation for effective problem solving and decision making. It will help you get the most out of the tailored solutions you're going to read about in subsequent chapters. And it can protect your health and welfare just as understanding blood sugar regulation does for those managing a chronic disease like diabetes.

Here are some ways that a solid understanding of OCD will help you navigate it and enjoy a better quality of life:

• **Effective, personalized decision making:** By understanding how OCD operates, you'll be able to identify quick and easy solutions that have a lasting impact, rather than repeatedly relying on temporary fixes that quickly lose their effectiveness. You'll also be able to tailor the strategies in this book to your particular needs.

7

- **Building empathy, support, and collaboration:** When you have accurate information, you'll be better able to educate others who can provide empathy, support, and encouragement. You'll also be able to combat misconceptions, stand up for yourself, and reduce stigma, resulting in a more supportive and understanding atmosphere.

- **Avoiding unintended consequences:** Solutions that are not based on a solid understanding of OCD can inadvertently create new challenges or exacerbate existing ones, such as harm to a relationship or difficulties at work.

- **Personal growth:** Understanding the challenges that OCD presents increases your self-awareness and self-acceptance. This will make you more resilient and better able to tackle problems, acquire resources, and gather advice. And if you've been wary of seeking treatment, perhaps you'll be encouraged to give it a try. (If so, see Chapter 12.)

What Is OCD?

As defined by the American Psychiatric Association, and as shown in the chart below, OCD involves two components. First, nonsensical but upsetting thoughts, ideas, mental images, and doubts—called *obsessions*—intrude into your mind (often triggered by something in the environment) even though you don't want them there. Your obsessions

Obsessions and emotional distress	Compulsions and avoidance to control the obsessions and distress
• Senseless intrusive unwanted thoughts, doubts, and images that keep recurring despite trying everything to get rid of them • Anxiety, fear, and uncertainty provoked by obsessions	• Compulsive behaviors, mental rituals, avoidance • Provide short-term escape from obsessional thoughts • Become ingrained patterns that take up time and interfere with life

might seem illogical on the one hand, but on the other hand they might have a true-to-life quality that's hard to ignore. That's why they provoke distress in the form of anxiety, fear, doubt, disgust, shame, or uncertainty that something bad might happen or has already happened. Second, because obsessions are upsetting, you try different ways to get rid of them; but the harder you try to control these thoughts and feelings, the more intense they seem to become.

The themes of obsessions can be about virtually anything, but they often focus on:

- Contamination from dirt, germs, or toxins
- Responsibility for making improbable mistakes
- Being at fault for causing (or not doing enough to prevent) bad luck, disasters, and physical or emotional harm
- Unwanted thoughts or images of violence or sex
- Unwanted thoughts of acting on impulses to say or do something cruel or hurtful
- Fears of becoming someone you are not (such as a child molester)
- Unwelcome ideas related to religion, sin, and morality
- Intrusive ideas of an existential nature that can never be fully resolved or answered (such as about the meaning of life)
- The feeling that something is "not just right" unless it's ordered or arranged a certain way

Your particular obsessions likely concern the very things you care about most deeply. If you have obsessions about contamination, it's likely you strongly value cleanliness. People who obsess over improbable mistakes are usually the most conscientious folks. And if you have obsessional thoughts about cruel, blasphemous, or dishonest acts, you're likely someone who takes matters of justice, morality, or religion very seriously. In other words, you're the last person who would actually act on these kinds of unwanted thoughts.

Finally, obsessions make you feel like you've got to do whatever you can to dismiss the thoughts, reduce the distress, and prevent or protect yourself and others from disaster.

Compulsions (sometimes called *compulsive rituals*) and *avoidance* of fear triggers are the kinds of behavior patterns you use to cope with obsessions, restore a feeling of safety and certainty, and reduce anxiety. Just about any behavior pattern can become a compulsion if it is intended to lessen obsessional fear, yet the most common ones are:

- Excessive washing or cleaning or using other means to sanitize
- Repeated checking
- Seeking reassurance from others
- Mental rituals (performed entirely in your head) such as excessive praying, overanalyzing situations, and thinking a "good" thought to suppress or replace a "bad" one
- Ordering and arranging things
- Repeating routine behaviors such as touching the door or switching the lights off and on

There are two key points here:

1. *Obsessions are unwanted thoughts that **provoke** fear, uncertainty, and discomfort.*
2. *Compulsive rituals, mental rituals, and avoidance are attempts to **reduce** the distress associated with obsessional thoughts.*

For many people, when they think of OCD they immediately think of extreme tidiness and perfectionism. But OCD can manifest in numerous ways that go beyond a preference for neatness. On a similar note, OCD is not just a personality quirk or a personal preference. It is a clinically recognized mental health disorder that significantly impacts daily life and well-being.

Indeed the symptoms of OCD cast a long shadow and trigger extensive "collateral damage" across many important domains of life. As if the interference and emotional pain resulting directly from obsessions and compulsions isn't enough, these symptoms also have ripple effects that disrupt your day-to-day routine and linger even after successful treatment. That's because therapies are mostly focused on reducing obsessions and compulsions per se and less on helping you solve problems that are related to OCD yet outside the realm of these symptoms such as:

- Self-stigma and shame
- Difficulties managing time and staying organized
- Trouble communicating with others about OCD
- Struggles in navigating work or school
- Strained relationships with family and friends
- Complications with dating and intimate relationships

Finally, there are times in life, and certain circumstances, that cause us more than the usual stress. For example, a loved one has fallen ill or passed away, or you've lost a job or close relationship. In times like these, even if you've had successful treatment and are managing your OCD symptoms well, you're likely to see an uptick in obsessions and compulsions. All of these consequences and impacts of OCD are why you may need help in addition to what even the most effective OCD treatments can offer. This book provides you with exactly that.

How OCD Gets You Stuck in a Vicious Cycle

Have you tried to put a stop to OCD by logically analyzing your intrusive thoughts and fears, by attempting to dismiss or suppress obsessions, or by promising yourself (and others) that you'll cease your compulsive rituals? After all, these seem like reasonable strategies for stopping bizarre, embarrassing, and time-consuming thoughts and behaviors. But if you're like most people with OCD, you know that these strategies don't work—at least not as long-term solutions. In fact, they only end up adding fuel to the fire and getting you stuck in a vicious cycle that's extremely difficult to get out of once you're trapped within.

It's important to thoroughly understand how this cycle operates— as a complex interplay of thoughts, emotions, and behaviors—so you'll know why it is that the more you try to fight or reason with obsessions, the *more* powerful they become, and why it's so difficult to just stop your rituals by sheer force of will. It will also help you get the most out of what's in this book because you'll understand how and where strategies *can* be applied and where or when they *won't* work. So, here's how it all unfolds.

Everyday Unwanted Thoughts

The vicious cycle begins with common everyday unwanted intrusive thoughts. You might not realize it, but these kinds of thoughts are a natural part of the human experience whether or not someone has OCD. They can range from fleeting concerns to very bizarre or unsettling ideas, images, and doubts. They might come to mind spontaneously or be triggered by something in the environment. Take Ariana, for example, who adores her beautiful newborn son but gets unwanted thoughts of throwing the infant down the stairs every time she uses a staircase. Most people just brush off these kinds of thoughts because they don't align with their core beliefs or values; therefore, the thoughts don't cause much distress or disruption. However, if you have OCD, the process goes very differently and leads to the development of obsessions.

Faulty Beliefs and Misinterpretations

People with OCD hold certain mistaken beliefs and assumptions such as the tendency to overestimate risk and danger, the notion that even senseless or bizarre unwanted thoughts are personally significant and threatening, and the belief that feelings like anxiety and uncertainty are intolerable. If you hold these types of faulty beliefs, then when benign unwanted intrusive thoughts spring to mind—especially thoughts that clash with your personal values—they'll grab your attention and trigger heightened levels of anxiety, discomfort, and doubt.

Ariana held the belief that *only bad people have thoughts about doing bad things.* So it's not surprising that the benign thoughts about harming her baby became "sticky," and she soon found herself worrying about them more and more. As the importance of these intrusive thoughts grew, she started to (mis)interpret their mere presence as an indicator that something was terribly wrong. She catastrophized the implications of her thoughts and became fearful that having them was a sign of an inherent personality flaw: *What if I'm dangerous and act on these thoughts!?*

Avoidance and Compulsions Form a Negative Reinforcement Loop

Although avoidance and compulsive rituals sometimes relieve anxiety in the short run, they're an important ingredient in the vicious cycle of OCD because over time they actually *strengthen* the connection between the intrusive thought and the perceived threat. Here's how:

First, avoidance and rituals keep you from self-correcting the faulty beliefs and appraisals just described. Ariana avoided carrying her baby near staircases as much as possible, and if she couldn't avoid them, she would repeat special phrases and prayers over and over to herself (mental rituals) to neutralize the unwanted thoughts and make her feel safer. But while these coping strategies reduced her distress in the moment, they kept her from realizing that she wasn't going to throw her son down the stairs anyway. In other words, when nothing bad happened, Ariana incorrectly attributed keeping her baby safe to her rituals rather than to the fact that she loved her baby and had no intention of harming him. As a result, she continued to believe that her intrusive thoughts meant that something was wrong. Soon one round of rituals didn't do the job and several rounds had to be made. Do you see how avoidance and rituals keep the vicious cycle going?

Avoidance and rituals also prompt more unwanted intrusive thoughts, which is similar to what happens if you look at your alarm clock when you're having trouble falling asleep. You may know that watching the clock is the worst thing you can do if you have insomnia because it only reminds you of how much sleep you're not getting. It makes you more stressed about trying to get to sleep, which makes you less likely to actually fall asleep. Similarly, as rituals grow over time, you become more and more preoccupied with your upsetting thoughts because they're the reasons you're doing the rituals in the first place. The more Ariana used rituals to cope with her thoughts and fears, the more she thought about the evil things she could do to her infant.

It's the same with trying to dismiss or suppress thoughts. The harder you work to *not* think about something, the more you'll think about it. Try an experiment: Think about anything in the world *except a white bear.* What's the first thought that comes to mind? Likely a white bear. Similarly, when you try to avoid or dismiss unwanted intrusive thoughts, they just reoccur—it's just another way you can get caught in the vicious cycle of OCD.

What's worse is that because rituals, avoidance, and thought suppression sometimes give you *temporary* relief, a negative reinforcement loop is established, and you get drawn into using these unhelpful strategies again and again hoping that they'll finally bring lasting relief. But what only happens is that these behaviors snowball, occupying more and more space in your life and provoking more and more intrusive thoughts. Maybe you spend hours ritualizing each day or avoiding certain situations even though doing so is very inconvenient. It's these behavior patterns that are most responsible for disruptions in your work or school life, your relationships, personal health and hygiene, and your leisure time.

Escalation into Obsessions

As the negative reinforcement loop strengthens, the intrusive thoughts gain power and transform into obsessions. They become more frequent, intense, and harder to dismiss. Your attempts to suppress or control them, reason with them, and gain reassurance become increasingly futile, leading to heightened distress and preoccupation. Not only that, struggles to manage the obsessions through avoidance and compulsions further solidify their hold on your psyche. The obsessions intrude into different parts of your life, disrupting your concentration, social activities, and leisure time. As this process played out for Ariana, her life became more and more about struggling with obsessional thoughts and less and less about spending quality time with her baby.

The diagram on the facing page shows the factors just described and how they form a self-perpetuating vicious loop. This cycle explains why you can't just simply "stop obsessing" and why it's not merely a lack of willpower or self-discipline that's keeping you from stopping your rituals. There's an intricate interaction of factors at play that makes

THE VICIOUS CYCLE OF OCD

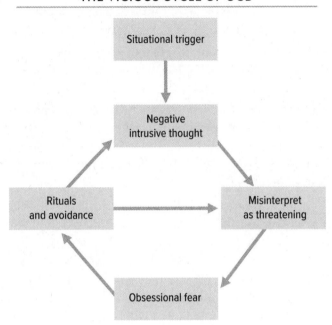

OCD difficult to overcome. The best way of breaking free from the cycle is by pursuing professional help. But even if you're not undergoing treatment, or if you're still experiencing OCD symptoms despite having tried treatment, understanding the cycle will prepare you to use the strategies in this book to improve your well-being, increase your productivity at work or school, and communicate clearly with others about OCD to build a network of support.

How Do You Reduce OCD Symptoms?

The OCD cycle provides a road map for therapists, informing them of how to intervene (and how *not* to intervene) to successfully reduce obsessions and compulsions. For example, since unwanted intrusive thoughts are ordinary benign experiences, there's no value in trying to help people with OCD dismiss their obsessions. Think back to the white bear experiment. Any "treatment" that tries to teach you to control or suppress intrusive thoughts (like snapping a rubber band on your wrist whenever obsessions show up) can't be very effective. Similarly, there's no reason to think that taking you back to your childhood or probing your subconscious mind in search of the ultimate cause of OCD will be helpful in breaking free of the vicious cycle.

What the vicious cycle *does* indicate is that two changes are necessary if you're going to successfully reduce OCD symptoms:

1. You must correct the faulty beliefs and misinterpretations that lead to obsessions.

2. You must eliminate avoidance and rituals because they reinforce obsessional fear.

The most effective way to make these changes is by using a treatment called exposure and response prevention (ERP). ERP, which is a form of cognitive-behavioral therapy (CBT), is backed by decades of research showing that it reduces OCD symptoms by 60–70% on average when implemented correctly. There are also medications that can be helpful for OCD called selective serotonin reuptake inhibitors (or SSRIs). The SSRIs, however, result in only a 20–40% symptom reduction on average, which is why they are best used in combination with ERP. Chapter 12 provides strategies for getting the most out of treatment—especially ERP—should you decide to try it. For now, let's focus on how ERP breaks the OCD cycle, why ERP isn't for everyone, and what you can do about OCD symptoms in case you haven't tried it, or you have but it hasn't delivered the desired results.

What Is ERP?

ERP is a practical and skills-based approach to psychotherapy that aims to help you learn that obsessional fears are groundless and that compulsive rituals are not necessary for dealing with anxiety and uncertainty or for preventing feared outcomes. The technique of *exposure* involves deliberately confronting the situations, objects, and intrusive thoughts that provoke obsessional fear. The exposure is usually done gradually, starting with less anxiety-provoking situations and thoughts and progressing to more challenging ones with the coaching and support of your therapist. Most often, exposure occurs in real life, meaning that you engage directly with the situation or stimulus. Ariana, for example, might practice carrying her infant up and down stairs to learn that doing so is perfectly safe. Exposure may also occur in imagination to help you engage with obsessional thoughts. For example, Ariana would be coached to deliberately think the very thoughts about harming her son that she had been trying to push away. The purpose of imaginal exposure is to help you learn that unwanted thoughts are also not signs of danger. Finally, *response prevention* involves practice in refraining from the usual compulsive rituals that you would use to reduce anxiety. Ariana, for example, would be helped to resist the urges to repeat prayers and phrases.

How Does ERP Work?

If ERP sounds like a challenge, that's because it is. However, the challenge might not seem as formidable when you understand why these techniques are so effective in reducing obsessions and compulsions. The central idea is that ERP helps you learn that (1) your feared situations and intrusive thoughts are not as dangerous as you imagine and (2) you can manage anxiety, doubt, and other negative emotions better than you think. You also learn that the distress you experience is only temporary, so you don't need to spend your time doing rituals to remove anxiety. Of course, you could merely *discuss* these issues with a therapist, but ERP provides real-life experiential evidence, which is more convincing and longer lasting than what can be achieved from just talking. Experience is simply the best teacher.

As you confront the intrusive thoughts and triggers, they become less scary, and urges to perform compulsions gradually diminish. That's because confronting something that isn't actually dangerous results in *habituation*. ERP also helps you put your fears to the test, including your fear that you wouldn't be able to handle the anxiety, doubt, and other forms of emotional distress. When ERP is done correctly and frequently, it gives you valuable and long-lasting learning experiences that you can't get if you are doing avoidance and rituals.

ERP Is Not for Everyone

But ERP has pros and cons. Although it can be extremely helpful and its effects can be long-lasting, you have to deliberately face the same situations you've been trying to avoid. Not only that, ERP is not effective for everyone, due to individual differences in the severity and nature of OCD symptoms, comorbid conditions (like severe depression or ADHD), or difficulties in fully engaging with the therapy itself. And even when ERP does help, its effects are often limited to OCD symptoms themselves. This means that difficulties in other areas of your life that have been impacted by OCD, such as your self-esteem, social functioning, and work satisfaction, might not be addressed completely.

Accordingly, for a variety of reasons, you may have passed on this treatment, and that's understandable. Facing feared situations without doing rituals might seem like too great a risk to take right now. Perhaps you're concerned about experiencing "too much" anxiety. You might also feel strongly that your obsessions are realistic, and your rituals are worthwhile, so it's just not worth changing your routine. For instance, it made perfect sense to Ariana to do mental rituals when carrying her child on the stairs. To her, these compulsions kept her baby safe. As long as she'd been doing them, she never harmed her child. So, she figured, *why risk it?*

Whether you've steered clear of ERP altogether, tried it and discontinued it midstream, or completed it but didn't get the improvement you'd hoped for, please know that many others are in the same boat. And even if ERP (or another treatment approach) improved your OCD symptoms but didn't completely address how OCD has interfered with your life, I've got your back. In this book I introduce you to lots of strategies and resources to help you find the right path for living a rich and meaningful life.

Congratulations! You now have the essential knowledge about OCD needed to fully benefit from the strategies in this book and make living with this disorder easier and more satisfying—even if existing treatments have failed you in one way or another. Many people with

OCD harbor shame and self-stigma about their disorder. Many feel guilty that OCD is burdensome to the people in their lives, such as their family and friends. Chapter 2 addresses these apprehensions and provides strategies for how to become more self-compassionate. I'll meet you there!

Practical Steps for Living Well: Charting a Path

Remember the power of your own brain:

- Fighting OCD doesn't help, but outwitting it can.
- Intrusive thoughts are normal, but you're in charge of how you respond to them.

Favor long-term solutions over temporary patches:

- Obeying OCD only makes it stronger.
- Less pain in single moments doesn't stop the pain from coming back.

Keep your eye on the prize: living well with OCD:

- Consider how quieting OCD through ERP could improve your quality of life.
- Be realistic with yourself about how much time you're losing on obsessions and compulsions.

2

replacing shame and guilt with self-compassion

The experience of OCD isn't just the relentless cycle of obsessions and compulsions described in Chapter 1. It's also an emotional journey with feelings of guilt and shame coming along for the ride. These feelings arise when you see yourself as a burden to those around you, judge yourself harshly, and think others are judging you just as severely. And not only do these thoughts and feelings compound the distress of obsessional fear; they also create added barriers to productive functioning and keep you from seeking help and support. In this chapter you'll learn strategies for combating shame and guilt so you can disentangle your self-worth from OCD symptoms. Specifically, you'll learn to cultivate self-compassion, recognize your personal values and strengths, and find fulfillment beyond the constraints of OCD. The first step is understanding that shame and guilt are a common part of having OCD.

Meet the Bad Guys: Shame and Guilt

Shame is a painful sense of humiliation or distress that's triggered when we perceive ourselves as flawed or inadequate. It's the feeling that *I am bad,* and it's especially upsetting because it targets your self-worth and can lead to its own cycle of self-criticism, avoidance of enjoyable activities, depression, more self-criticism, and so on. As an example, Nora overheard some of her friends mockingly describe another coworker as "crazy" because she's "so OCD" about tidiness. This made Nora feel embarrassed and worried that her own OCD would be seen as a joke. Would her friends also think she was crazy if they knew she had OCD? In addition to feelings of inadequacy and inferiority, shame can keep you from seeking professional help, fearing judgment from health care providers or thinking they won't take your problem seriously.

Guilt is the feeling that you've either done something you *shouldn't* have or not done something you *should* have. Take Ethan, whose OCD centers around a need for symmetry and order. His partner, Maya, is understanding but doesn't always remember to keep things the way Ethan likes. One day Ethan comes home to find that Maya's rearranged the living room furniture. In a fit of anxiety, he snaps at her and calls her selfish and uncaring. Later, when his anxiety subsides, he reflects on his outburst and understands that Maya had only been trying to refresh their living space. He feels a deep sense of guilt, realizing that his anger, driven by OCD, hurt someone he loves. Like many people with OCD, Ethan grapples with shame and regret over the emotional toll his disorder is taking on those around him.

Meet the Good Guys: Self-Compassion and Self-Acceptance

Self-compassion means treating yourself with the same kindness and understanding as you would offer a dear friend. It's about recognizing that everyone, including you, is deserving of empathy and kindheartedness, regardless of their challenges. When moments of shame and guilt arise, instead of succumbing to self-criticism, you can ask, "How can I support and care for myself right now?" By consistently choosing self-compassion over shame and guilt, you can foster a more nurturing, understanding relationship with yourself, aiding in the overall journey of managing and living well with OCD.

A related concept is *self-acceptance,* which involves recognizing and embracing all facets of yourself, including your strengths and weaknesses. For someone with OCD, self-acceptance means acknowledging the presence of the disorder without judging yourself for having it. It's a conscious effort to avoid viewing OCD as a character flaw, and instead understand that your value as a person isn't diminished by having this disorder.

While these concepts overlap, they represent different aspects of personal growth. Self-compassion offers a nurturing approach, while self-acceptance is about embracing yourself. You need both to summon the resilience that's required to navigate life with OCD. They help you bounce back from adversity, adapt in the face of challenges, and maintain confidence when you encounter setbacks. The rest of this chapter includes exercises and strategies to promote self-compassion and self-acceptance. They'll help you maximize your potential in the following ways:

• **Boosting your self-image:** You'll repair any damage that OCD has done to your self-image and allow yourself to see your strengths, talents, and capabilities. You'll start to see OCD as just one aspect of your multifaceted identity.

• **Increasing resilience:** You'll gain the confidence that you can manage whatever OCD throws at you. It won't always be easy, but you'll reduce the impact of obsessions and compulsions.

• **Strengthening relationships:** You'll be in a better frame of mind to communicate openly with others about your struggles (using strategies covered in later chapters). This openness leads to a stronger support network and more meaningful relationships.

• **Reducing anxiety:** By accepting and understanding that OCD is only a part of you—not your whole identity—you'll approach your symptoms with a calmer mind-set.

• **Setting realistic expectations:** You'll be able to set realistic daily goals for yourself, acknowledging that some days might be harder than others, but that doesn't diminish your overall progress or worth.

Shattering the Shackles of Shame and Guilt

Shame and guilt (along with *self-stigma,* which means accepting negative stereotypes about OCD) can hinder well-being. But your struggles don't define you. Your inherent worth as a person isn't based on your challenges, successes, or society's views. Everyone has unique strengths and struggles. Instead of letting OCD dictate your self-worth, recognize your diverse strengths and qualities aside from this disorder. This broader perspective can foster self-acceptance without dismissing the issues that OCD brings.

Beyond OCD: Discovering Your True Self

Try this exercise to gain a deeper understanding and appreciation of yourself beyond the confines of OCD. The goal is to develop a more holistic self-concept that emphasizes your unique qualities, strengths, and experiences, helping you see that while OCD is a part of your life, it isn't your entire identity.

You'll need a comfortable space free from distractions, something to write with, and a journal or a few sheets of paper. I encourage you to truly immerse yourself in this exercise, as well as the others in the book. There is a wealth of tools here, but it's through your heartfelt engagement with the exercises and strategies that you'll experience the most profound transformations.

To prepare, sit back, close your eyes, and take a few deep breaths. Think of yourself as a multifaceted diamond. OCD might be one facet of this diamond, but there are many other sides and angles that make you who you are.

1. *Now ask yourself: Who am I beyond my OCD?*

2. *Next, start writing down qualities about yourself that aren't related to OCD.* These qualities can be roles you play (such as parent, friend, teammate, teacher, artist, nature lover), qualities you possess (such as gentle, curious, attractive), or experiences you cherish (such as taking a walk on a crisp day or hearing a certain song). Then think about moments in your life when you felt proud, accomplished, or fulfilled.

Those moments could be the times when you overcame a challenge, completed a project, gave a recital, helped your team win a game, graduated from school, reached a relationship milestone, or had a personal growth moment. Also recall the feedback you've received from others about your strengths and qualities. Write a few lines describing these occasions and what they were like for you.

3. *Next, ask yourself: What are the things I love doing?* They could be hobbies, activities, or other interests. Jot down anything that brings you joy or ignites your passion. Picture a day where OCD doesn't play a dominant role. What would you do? Who would you spend it with? How would you feel? Write down this visualization in detail.

4. *Next, briefly note how OCD affects your life.* Remember, the objective of this exercise is not to minimize the impact of OCD but to place it in the larger context of who you are.

5. *Now use what you've written so far to compose five to ten affirmations about yourself.* Affirmations are positive, clear statements meant to inspire and motivate you. They're typically phrased in the present tense and aim to promote a sense of confidence. Here are some examples from people with whom I've used this exercise:

- *I embrace all parts of myself, understanding that OCD is just one part of me.*
- *I am multifaceted, I have skills and interests, and I am unique.*
- *I've survived 100% of my worst days with OCD. Every challenge makes me stronger.*
- *My worth is not determined by my thoughts or my rituals.*
- *I am deserving of love, understanding, and compassion, regardless of my OCD.*
- *I am not alone; I have people in my life who understand and support me.*

6. *Finally, take some time to read out loud everything you've written.* Say the words confidently, let them sink in, and feel the emotions they elicit. It's okay if speaking out loud feels a bit awkward or forced at first; with time and practice it becomes more natural. Introduce your affirmations into your daily routine. For instance, you could say the words while looking at yourself in the mirror or during a quiet moment.

The morning is an especially good time, as it can help you set a self-compassionate tone for the rest of the day.

Do you find it difficult to believe your affirmations? That's normal too, especially when you start out. But don't give up—give the exercise time and be patient. Try framing your affirmations as goals, such as *I'm working on becoming more confident every day*. Also remember that the objective is not to deny the reality of OCD or make it seem like everything is all rainbows and unicorns! It's to empower yourself in managing OCD and recognizing your worth beyond it. With consistent practice the exercise can be a powerful tool in cultivating a self-accepting mind-set. Our brains have a feature known as *neuroplasticity,* which is the ability to form new pathways. When we repeat affirmations, we create fresh neural connections, slowly eroding the older ones associated with shame and guilt. But this process can take some time.

What Do You Want Your Life to Be About?

It's a profound question, yet vital to consider as you journey toward self-acceptance and navigate the complexities of OCD. The principles and ideals that provide guidance, purpose, and direction in your life are called *core values*. Some examples include maintaining physical health, strong family ties, honesty, financial independence, religious devotion, social justice, and occupational or academic achievement. Taking time to clarify your values helps you separate yourself from OCD. It's also a form of self-affirmation that paves the way to self-acceptance. In the next exercise you'll define what's meaningful to you across different life domains so you can live in alignment with your values despite obsessions, anxiety, and compulsions.

Aligning with Your Core Values

Derived from ACT (acceptance and commitment therapy), the Values Target is a visual tool that helps you identify and connect with your core values. It also allows you to gauge how you're adhering to these values in the face of OCD's challenges. I introduce this tool to my patients, assisting them in clarifying their genuine priorities beyond obsessions and compulsions. To undertake this exercise, you'll need a large sheet of paper or whiteboard, a pen or marker, and a printed or drawn target on the paper/board, like Tanya's example below. Tanya's OCD concerned obsessional thoughts of a sexual, violent, and blasphemous nature along with reassurance-seeking compulsions.

Begin by listing your core values in these four areas of life: (1) work or education, (2) personal growth and health, (3) relationships, and (4) leisure. Like what Tanya identified, these values should represent what truly matters to you; but let's distinguish between *values* and *goals* because they're often confused for one another. Goals are specific, tangible targets with a clear end point, like losing a set amount of weight or reading a certain number of books. Values, on the other hand, are principles, such as honesty or compassion, that provide a

TANYA'S VALUES TARGET

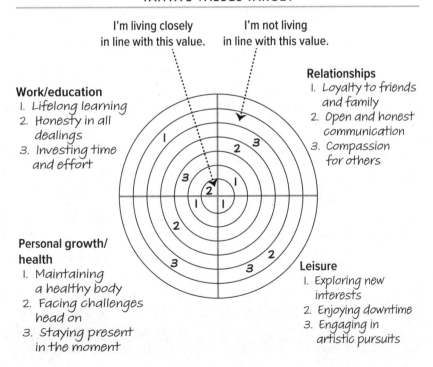

I'm living closely in line with this value.   **I'm not living in line with this value.**

Work/education
1. Lifelong learning
2. Honesty in all dealings
3. Investing time and effort

Relationships
1. Loyalty to friends and family
2. Open and honest communication
3. Compassion for others

Personal growth/ health
1. Maintaining a healthy body
2. Facing challenges head on
3. Staying present in the moment

Leisure
1. Exploring new interests
2. Enjoying downtime
3. Engaging in artistic pursuits

sense of purpose and direction for the decisions you make in your life. We don't "reach" values the way we reach goals; we just continue to live in line with our values.

As Tanya did, label each quadrant of your target with one of the life domains and number each value you identified. Then think carefully about how much you are living in line with each value and mark the number of the value on the target. The more your actions are consistent with that value, the closer you can put the corresponding number to the center (the bull's-eye). Once you've finished, take in the big picture and ask yourself: Which areas of my life are closely aligned with my values? Which ones are farther away? For areas that are farther from the bull's-eye, recognize the role that OCD might be playing in keeping you from being attuned to those values.

For example, Tanya's Values Target shows that despite having OCD, she was living fully in line with her values of honesty, loyalty, exploring new interests, and taking care of her body. On the other hand, she was struggling with continuing her education, remaining in the moment during activities, enjoying leisure time and artistic pursuits, and communicating and empathizing with others. Upon reflection, she realized she was having trouble living in accordance with these values because OCD made it hard for her to finish college, her intrusive thoughts were too distracting, she was too exhausted from fighting her obsessions to enjoy leisure and create art, and her continual quest for reassurance from family members strained these relationships.

Moving toward the Bull's-Eye

For areas where you aim to align more with your values, set small, actionable goals or intentions. For example, Tanya decided she would learn and practice mindfulness skills (which you'll read about in Chapter 12) to help her stay present and in the moment during pleasurable activities, especially during her leisure time. Maybe your OCD symptoms interfere with spending quality time with loved ones. If so, you could set aside 20 minutes a day to spend with your family without allowing rituals to get in the way. Once you've set your intentions, commit to taking small steps. Don't aim for immediate perfection, but for gradual movement toward the bull's-eye. Finally, I recommend returning to your Values Target on a regular basis—perhaps every 3–6 months—to reassess where you stand, celebrate areas where you've moved closer to your core values, and readjust your plan as necessary. Speaking of celebrating successes . . .

Celebrating Success and Resilience

I find that people with OCD tend to underestimate their own courage and resilience. If facing a daily barrage of intrusive thoughts, triggers, and emotional turbulence is not the epitome of toughness, I'm not sure what is. Yet you probably don't give yourself the credit you deserve for this inner fortitude. Acknowledging your strength and resilience is another way to replace guilt and shame with self-compassion and self-acceptance. To do this, you've got to make every victory—even the small ones—count, from shaving a few minutes off your rituals to driving past that cemetery you've been avoiding. Learning to recognize and reinforce your resilience will help you cultivate confidence, counteract negative self-talk, and decrease the power of OCD. Here are some strategies to help you do so.

Charting Resilience

Think about a recent instance when you showed resilience in the face of OCD—that is, when you displayed toughness and the ability to recover quickly from adversity. Maybe you resisted a compulsion, confronted a fear, or even identified an intrusive thought as OCD driven. Document this instance in your journal, noting the situation, your feelings and thoughts, coping strategy, and the outcome. Take some time to reflect on your resilience. Write down how you felt afterward. Were you proud or empowered? Did this experience change your approach the next time you were in a similar situation? Finally, write an affirmation based on your experience, such as "I have the strength to face my fears and resist my compulsions." Regularly log such moments of resilience, accumulating a collection of reminders of your strength and ability to cope with OCD.

It's okay if your moment of resilience seems minor; any act of resilience highlights your strength. If pinpointing such a moment proves difficult, don't be discouraged. Instead, aim to recognize such moments moving forward—such a commitment itself is a form of resilience.

This exercise not only highlights your strength against OCD but also chronicles your progress. Looking back on these moments can be uplifting and empowering, especially during rough times. To take this strategy a step further, create a tangible way to track acts of resilience. For example, add a marble to a glass jar each time you resist a compulsion. Display the jar prominently so it becomes a constant reminder of your commitment to resilience (and take pride in sharing its significance with curious observers).

Seeking Positive Feedback

Another effective way to understand your resilience is to ask others to tell you when they notice you tackling challenges such as facing a situation you typically avoid, handling anxiety, or resisting compulsions. By actively seeking this kind of feedback, you'll not only achieve a clearer understanding of your own accomplishments but also foster deeper connections with those who support you. Their perspectives can shed light on areas of your resilience and personal growth you tend to overlook, bolstering your confidence and inner fortitude on your way to living well.

Begin by choosing a handful of trusted family members or close friends whom you trust to provide genuine feedback. Let them know you're looking to better appreciate the strengths they see in you, especially regarding your resilience against OCD. To ensure a focused and open conversation, schedule a dedicated time to chat face-to-face, over the phone, or through a virtual platform.

Plan your questions in advance before seeking feedback. You'll get the most information when you ask *open-ended* questions: "How have you noticed changes in how I manage OCD?" "Tell me about a time when I showed resilience or strength against OCD," and "What are my strengths that I overlook?" Avoid closed-ended questions like "Do I have any strengths?" because they tend to yield basic yes/no answers. Document the key points from these conversations so you can revisit and reflect on them later. Finally, always show your appreciation to those you converse with, valuing their time and unique insights.

Take time to reflect on the positive feedback you've gathered, focusing on the qualities other people see in you. Regularly review your notes as a reminder of your strengths and the progress you've made. This practice strengthens your resolve to thrive despite OCD.

Rewarding Resilience

Rewarding your resilience is a powerful way to strengthen your positive coping strategies and turn guilt and shame into self-compassion. Start by creating a list of fun and meaningful rewards. They could range from self-care activities and favorite treats to buying a desired item or indulging in a favorite hobby. Link each act of resilience to a reward, but make sure the significance of the reward matches the scale of your achievement, with bigger rewards for overcoming more significant challenges. As you enjoy your reward, savor the moment and reflect on your achievement. Deeply acknowledging your growth and accomplishments encourages you to repeat the positive behavior in the future. Periodically refresh your reward list to keep the exercise challenging.

Embracing Identity beyond OCD

Does OCD cast a shadow on other parts of your identity? Shifting your perspective from shame to self-acceptance allows you to embrace an identity beyond OCD. This shift involves delving into and rejuvenating your interests and passions. You've already identified your values and noticed your resilience. Now it's time to align your actions with what resonates deeply with you and leverage your inner strengths. Engaging in activities that bring you joy and fulfillment can counteract the challenges posed by OCD, nurturing a sense of well-being and purpose. As you explore the following suggestions, think about your core values and where your inherent strengths lie. Let your insights from this chapter help you decide on next steps.

Pursue Your Passions

Look for activities or causes that genuinely excite you to add a fresh sense of purpose to your life and carve out spaces for energy and enjoyment beyond the constraints of OCD. A deep dive into something you love also anchors your mind, making it harder for unwanted obsessional thoughts to take center stage. What's more, pursuing hobbies and supporting causes often lead to meeting people with mutual interests. These connections help forge relationships that aren't centered around OCD, broadening your social horizons and offering camaraderie in both challenging times and moments of achievement.

Explore New Hobbies

Maybe you're struggling to find a passion or just looking for something new. Start by thinking about what genuinely excites or intrigues you; maybe a newfound curiosity or something you've long cherished. Be mindful of potential OCD triggers and choose a hobby that feels comfortable and won't provoke distress. Instead of diving headfirst into something, gradually ease yourself in. For example, if you're interested in painting, start with simple sketches before investing in a full set of paints and canvases. Prioritize enjoyment over perfection. The journey is more important than the outcome.

Activities can be categorized into two types: *Structured* hobbies are those with a clear direction, such as knitting, reading, playing music, and building models. *Expressive* hobbies, on the other hand, are more free-form and fluid, like abstract painting, writing your own music, or playing a sport. They can help with venting pent-up emotions and breaking free from inflexibility. Joining a class or group can help you stay committed and enhance socialization, but make sure the group dynamics don't become a source of stress. You might initially prefer a solitary activity, seeking a group setting as your comfort grows. There are also numerous online platforms, from YouTube to specialized hobby forums, where you can learn new skills at your own pace. Social media can be a great place to start, especially if leaving the house or joining groups feels daunting. Ultimately, your chosen hobby should provide an opportunity for relaxation, creativity, and self-expression. You're looking for something to serve as a constructive outlet for redirecting energy, fostering a sense of accomplishment, and creating an identity apart from the confines of OCD.

Lend a Helping Hand

Lending a hand to others can be an enriching and transformative experience. It gives you a fresh perspective on your own challenges by revealing the universality of human struggles. By immersing yourself in acts of service, you not only find reprieve from the relentless cycle of obsessions and compulsions, but also discover a profound sense of purpose. This altruistic engagement acts as a reminder that even amid your battles with OCD, you have the capacity to make a positive impact on the world, reinforcing self-worth and cultivating a purpose that rises above the bounds of OCD. Here are some examples of ways you can help others:

- Help package or distribute food or prepare and serve meals to people who are food insecure
- Volunteer at shelters, helping with various tasks or organizing workshops
- Offer companionship to elderly people or provide help to connect them with loved ones
- Join conservation efforts such as tree-planting events or beach or park cleanups
- Assist students with their academic work or teach adult literacy classes
- Help care for animals or assist with adoptions
- Join organizations that offer relief during natural disasters
- Serve as a mentor for at-risk youth
- Volunteer at local museums, theaters, places of worship, or community art programs
- Organize drives that collect clothing for those in need

As you reflect on this chapter and engage in the exercises provided, remember that your journey with OCD is multilayered, encompassing not only obsessions and compulsions, but also internal struggles with guilt and shame. By highlighting your strengths, realigning with your personal values, recognizing your resilience, and embracing your full potential beyond OCD, you reduce the impact of shame and guilt. These strategies also foster self-compassion and self-acceptance, helping to clear the path to a more fulfilling and enriched life.

Practical Steps for Living Well:
Replacing Shame and Guilt with Self-Compassion

Cultivate self-compassion and self-acceptance:

- Be as kind and understanding to yourself as you would to a dear friend.
- Remember, having OCD doesn't diminish your value as a person.
- Introduce inspiring affirmations into your daily routine.

Follow your values:

- Identify your core values and recognize where OCD interferes with living by them.
- Use your resilience to align with your values despite your OCD symptoms.

Pursue your purpose:

- Engage in meaningful hobbies and other activities to focus on life beyond OCD.
- Volunteer for causes that matter to you to find a more rewarding purpose.

3

quieting obsessional fears and doubts

Because OCD is a chronic condition, whether or not you've undergone formal treatment and seen improvements, you'll still sometimes find yourself grappling with intrusive thoughts, fears, and doubts. Questions like "What if I made a terrible mistake?" and "How do I know I'm not going to act on some unwanted impulse?" may haunt your mind. Uncertainties like "What if God is upset with me?" and "What is my authentic identity and purpose?" might continue to crop up. Whether they come in the form of full-blown obsessions or as occasional lingering intrusions, these thoughts and fears are upsetting. They can undermine any progress you've achieved and cast a shadow over your day-to-day functioning.

In this chapter we'll delve into strategies for calming these obsessional thoughts and doubts. Although ERP is the most extensively studied treatment for OCD, research shows that other non-exposure-based approaches can also be excellent tools for navigating obsessions, uncertainties, and fears. Those approaches are the focus of this chapter. The strategies you'll find in the following pages are derived from acceptance and commitment therapy (ACT) and inference-based cognitive behavioral therapy (I-CBT). If you've hesitated to try ERP, these techniques offer an alternative for managing OCD symptoms. If you're already undergoing ERP (or have used it in the past) or taking medication, these strategies can supplement and enhance your treatment.

Changing Your Perspective on Obsessions

Think back to Chapter 1, where you learned that unwanted thoughts are not confined to people with OCD. This is a research-proven fact. Landmark studies dating back to the 1970s, along with a plethora of subsequent research, confirm that pretty much everyone sometimes grapples with unusual, upsetting, and even morally troubling thoughts, ideas, images, or doubts that intrude into consciousness and are incongruent with their personal values. Not only that, the *content* of these kinds of thoughts is similar whether you have OCD or not.

Read this list of intrusive thoughts and see if you can guess which ones are those of people with OCD and which ones are those of people without OCD:

- I could transmit germs to others and make them sick.
- What if I carry out the sexual behavior I'm thinking about.
- I could swerve into the opposite lane of traffic and cause a head-on collision.
- Is my zest for life strong enough that I won't commit suicide?
- What if I cause something disastrous by mistake?
- Did I forget to secure or turn off something before leaving the house?
- What if I did something that violates my moral or ethical principles?
- Could I be suffering from a severe illness?
- Is it OK if I looked in the direction of someone's private parts?
- I might harm someone I deeply care about.
- What if I've committed a spiritual or religious offense?
- What if I say something highly offensive or racist?

- Invisible germs and bacteria are covering my hands.
- I have blasphemous thoughts during prayer or in sacred places.

If you think these intrusive thoughts sound like classic obsessions of people with OCD, I don't blame you. However, I collected them from people who *don't* have OCD! This means that the problem in OCD isn't merely the *presence* of these thoughts. As you read in Chapter 1, how well you get through your daily life is determined by how you *respond* to such thoughts and not by whether you *have* them in the first place. Seeing your unwanted thoughts as facts and threats and then trying to dismiss or control them only lead to getting swept into the swirling vortex of OCD. So if you were hoping for techniques to forever banish your obsessional thoughts or replace them with positive ones, I'm sorry—that's simply not possible. But what I can do is offer you tools to shift your *perspective* on intrusive thoughts, enabling you to live a richer life even when they make an appearance.

Why Shift Perspective?

It's not that I don't *want* you to get rid of your obsessional thoughts. It would truly be amazing if there were a way to dismiss unwanted thoughts for good. But unfortunately, that's just not the way the brain works. Have you ever tried holding a fully inflated beach ball under water? It's futile—the more force you apply, the more it resists and pops back up. And that's what happens when you try to get rid of obsessional thoughts. Here's an exercise that demonstrates the futility of trying to dismiss thoughts.

1 3 5

Examine these three numbers. Memorizing them should be quick and easy. Once you feel confident that you've committed them to memory, cover them up or look away. Now try for 30 seconds to forget them. After that pause, can you recall what the numbers were? Were you able to completely erase them from your mind? When you're finished reading this chapter (or even this whole book), do you think you will have forgotten them?

The idea here is that once something has entered our conscious-ness, it often lingers. Do you believe this concept also applies to your obsessive thoughts? *You bet it does!* But if that's the case, how success-ful do you think attempts to forcefully remove them from your mind would be?

Let's try another exercise. Complete the following sentences:

- Birds of a feather _____.
- Don't cry over _____.
- Actions speak louder _____.

This exercise underscores the reality that efforts to control or expel thoughts are generally futile. It's just how the brain operates. We can't erase what's already there; and trying to do so only amplifies it, making it more intense. Now, if the contents of your mind were only benign sayings like the ones in this exercise, that would be one thing. But when thoughts venture into distressing, obsessive territories, it's a dif-ferent ball game. It can be disheartening to feel like your daily life is so controlled by your obsessions.

What if the solution lies not in dismissing or avoiding them, but in allowing them to show up while you alter how you relate to them?

Dropping the Rope

One tool to calm your struggle with obsessive thoughts is to imagine you're in a game of tug-of-war with a big, strong monster. This mon-ster symbolizes the obsessions and anxieties that your mind generates. The rope between you and the monster signifies your struggle to con-trol these unpleasant thoughts. A yawning chasm separates both of you, and it feels like the monster is trying to drag you into that abyss. You pull hard on the rope, and so does the monster. Neither of you has won the game, leaving you in a deadlock. Does it feel like you're trapped in this unwinnable situation?

But what if winning isn't the goal? What if there's another option, like simply letting go of the rope? The monster won't disappear, but your dynamic with it will shift. You end the struggle not because you've defeated the monster but because you recognize that battling it keeps you stuck in the conflict. When you let go and step back, you free yourself from a never-ending tug-of-war. Here are some strategies to help you let go of the rope and get unstuck from your obsessional thoughts when they crop up in your daily life.

GIVE IT A NAME

By labeling your obsessions for what they really are, you can gain a new perspective on them as mere unwanted thoughts, rather than definitive truths. So, when an obsessional thought comes to mind, don't just buy into it. Tag it by placing something in front of it. For example, say to yourself, *I'm having an unwanted thought about God* or *Ah, there's that recurring idea that I've left the door unlocked* or even, *Thanks, mind, for suggesting that there are dangerous germs on the doorknob.* You can even apply this technique to physical sensations, such as unwanted feelings in your groin that you might take to mean your sexual obsessions are accurate. When you actively identify intrusive obsessional thoughts for what they are, you reduce their power to control you.

TRANSFORM IT INTO AN OBJECT

You can also get unstuck from obsessions by turning them into tangible objects. Take an intrusive thought and imagine it outside your mind, as though you were observing it. Use the following questions to objectify the unwanted thought:

- What color would it be? What shape? How big or small?
- Would it be hot, cold, or somewhere in between? Would it be static or moving?
- What songs, books, or movies would it like? What sports teams? What would it do for a living?

Now reintroduce this visualized object into your awareness. By transforming the obsession into an object that you could observe, you empower yourself to "carry it with you" without letting it dictate your life.

CHANGE HOW YOU HEAR IT

You can also change your perspective on an obsession by altering how you *hear* it. Try saying the thought in the voice of a favorite comedian, cartoon character, celebrity, teacher, or someone you know with a distinctive accent or dialect. You'll be surprised at how easily the thought becomes less problematic when you hear it in a voice different from your own—like Elvis, Morgan Freeman, Arnold Schwarzenegger, or the late Queen Elizabeth of England. Make a recording of the voice and play it for yourself. You might also try articulating the thought very slowly or really fast. Try altering the pitch as well. Say it in a squeaky, high-pitched voice or in a deep, low tone.

MAKE IT MONOTONOUS

Obsessional thoughts are really just a string of syllables and words that carry meanings you've learned over time. That's why some words can trigger positive emotions while others may evoke negative ones. Consider the thought "What if I'm a murderer?" Now repeat the word *murderer* aloud a hundred times ("murderer, murderer, murderer, murderer . . . "). What do you notice about how the word starts to feel? When you hear a word repeatedly, it often loses its emotional charge and may even make it seem nonsensical or amusing. The next time an obsessional thought comes to mind, try this repetition strategy until the word's meaning starts to change. Did you ever think that "leaning into" an unwanted thought actually leads to "letting go"?

WRITE IT DOWN AND CARRY IT WITH YOU

Jot down your obsessional thoughts on index cards or pieces of paper and keep them with you in your wallet, purse, or pocket. From time to time, you'll stumble on these cards while reaching for something else. When you do, pause and read them. What's your next move? Most likely you'll just put them back and continue with whatever you were doing. Use this strategy for handling other obsessions when they surface. Acknowledge them, imagine they're written on one of your cards, and then proceed with your day. The cards (and the obsessional thoughts) literally remain in contact with you, but they don't have to interrupt your activities.

By consistently using these strategies, you'll train yourself to stop struggling with obsessional thoughts and more consistently let go of the metaphorical rope. In turn, you shift your viewpoint on intrusive thoughts, diminishing their influence on your everyday life.

Discrediting Your Obsessions

You can also quiet your obsessions by recognizing that they're based more on flawed logic than on reality and are more a product of your creativity and imagination than actual facts. Over 20 years ago, a tragic crime involving a mother methodically killing her young children attracted lots of media attention. This event naturally triggered intrusive thoughts and images about awful scenarios for even the most adoring of parents: *What if I did that to my child!?* Most people correctly reasoned that such intrusions had no basis in reality. They were confident that they'd never intentionally harm their kids, and so they went about their lives. But some people came to our OCD clinic extremely fearful that they might turn violent. Although the mother who killed her children had been diagnosed with postpartum psychosis—an extremely rare condition very different from OCD—this group was also engaging in avoidance and compulsive rituals to prevent what they perceived as imminent disaster. For these loving parents, it was as if their grasp of reality had become skewed, blurring the boundary between this tragic event and their trust in themselves.

A psychological term for this process is *inferential confusion,* which means mistaking hypothetical possibilities for reality. In other words, it's a process in which your feelings and behaviors are influenced by imagined ideas and stories rather than by concrete facts. I met Golda, the mother of two-year-old Ben, shortly after the tragic news story began to draw attention. Golda had been diagnosed with OCD as a teenager, but her obsessions were now focused squarely on the intrusive doubt that she might kill Ben just as the mentally ill mother had killed her own children. I'll use Golda's example to introduce a number of strategies drawn from I-CBT to help you manage your obsessions by recognizing and correcting inferential confusion.

Understanding the Logic behind Your Obsessions

There's a particular reasoning process that fuels obsessions, whether yours are focused on being contaminated, committing a mistake, causing bad luck, acting contrary to your principles, or anything else. In particular, you make inferences that danger is likely because of one or more of the following types of information (including examples of Golda's reasoning):

- Abstract facts (Some parents do harm their children; I'm about the same age as the mother who killed her children.)
- General rules (People who *do* bad things *think about it* first. So, I should avoid thinking about hurting Ben.)
- Hearsay (I keep hearing about violent behavior in the media.)
- Personal experiences (Sometimes I get angry with Ben and raise my voice.)
- It's possible (I *could* easily hurt Ben because I am much bigger and stronger than he is.)

Maybe you spot the problems with relying on these reasons to conclude that danger is present—we'll get to that shortly. The goal here is just to become aware of the reasoning process itself. Next you'll find some helpful strategies.

RECOGNIZING YOUR OBSESSIONAL REASONING

Begin by writing down your own obsessional doubts that provoke anxiety or compulsive rituals. Then, for each one, ask yourself why you think it could be true, even if it's extremely unlikely. For example, what are the reasons you believe you'll get sick from using a public bathroom? Why do you think you might have left the oven on? What makes you feel that you insulted someone or used a racial slur? Why do you believe you'll poison the food you're preparing for your family? Write down any justification you can think of in the categories of information presented in the previous list: abstract facts, general rules, hearsay, personal experience, and possibility. Use Golda's examples as a guide, but allow your OCD to "express itself."

WRITING YOUR OCD STORY

The reasons you use to justify your obsessional doubts form a story that makes your obsessions feel credible. This story influences how you feel and what you do in response to certain intrusive thoughts and situations. So next take the information you just wrote down and stitch it together to form your own "OCD story." Here's what Golda wrote:

> *I need to avoid thinking about killing Ben because these thoughts mean that I'm going to be the next homicidal mother. For one thing, I know there are some parents out there who murder their children. I'm also much bigger and stronger than Ben, so it's totally possible for me to overpower him. I'm also the same age as the woman who did this to her own children, and this similarity is very frightening. The worst thing is that sometimes, when Ben doesn't follow directions, I get angry with him and I've even screamed at him. So I'm definitely someone who is capable of losing myself in a fit of rage and killing my child.*

Can you see how, in the context of Golda's OCD story, thoughts about harming Ben and information about the tragic murders would provoke anxiety and avoidance behavior? Your story should similarly be able to explain why *you* feel anxious and engage in avoidance or rituals.

RECOGNIZING YOUR FEARED SELF

In I–CBT, your *feared self* is the person you're afraid you'll become if you don't do compulsive rituals or avoid feared situations. It's the antithesis (opposite) of who you really are. And it's the reason your obsessions aren't random.

You'll recognize your feared self in the recurring themes of your obsessional thoughts and doubts. Write down those themes. What similarities do they share? If they were true, what kind of person would you be? Presto . . . meet your feared self! In Golda's feared version of herself she was prone to anger, lacking in self-control, and highly susceptible to committing terrible acts despite her better judgment and will.

Now think about the evidence that supports this feared version of yourself. What convinces you that your obsessional doubts reveal something authentic about who you are? How do you justify believing that this is the person you'd become if you gave up your rituals?

Transforming the Narrative

Now that you've identified the reasons you use to justify your obsessional fears, let's scrutinize these arguments more carefully. Whatever your obsessional theme—contamination, mistakes, harm, sex, religion, existentialism, symmetry—all OCD stories contain the same holes in their logic: They don't align with direct facts or common sense, and they're not grounded in the present reality. Take Golda's story. She might sometimes become angry, yell, and have intrusive thoughts about killing her son; but these are only facts *about* reality without links to the here and now. There's no concrete information in the present moment that substantiates her fear that she will kill Ben. And her *internal* state of mind—her intentions and her judgment—certainly provides no basis for her feared self. Her OCD story is just that—*a story*. Nonetheless, it contains such personally meaningful and striking details that it influences her emotions and behavior (a fallacy psychologists call *emotional reasoning*).

The same fallacies are true of your OCD story (or stories). Learning to spot the logical inconsistencies is key to managing obsessions when they appear in your daily life. When you're able to do this, your narrative's credibility will melt away along with your fear and urges to do compulsive rituals. Here are some strategies to assist you.

REALITY CHECK

This strategy involves looking at your OCD story from someone else's point of view. First, try it with Golda's story by asking yourself what it would take to convince you that her story is valid. That is, what direct evidence from your senses—anything you can see, hear, taste, smell, or touch around you, along with your common sense—would make you concerned enough that you'd worry about her son's well-being? Here are some possibilities:

- You've seen that Golda exhibits apathy, hate, or hostility toward Ben.
- You saw Golda specifically threaten or attempt to harm Ben.
- Golda had a history of intentionally harming other people she says she loves.
- Golda consistently shows poor judgment, disregard, and negligence when it comes to caring for Ben.
- Common sense told you that parents often lie about how much they love their children.
- Common sense told you that parents go around acting on unwanted thoughts of harming their children.

Now contrast this with the justifications in Golda's OCD story. Do you see the differences? All the points provided here are specific and directly related to the context of the obsession (and they're *false!*). In contrast, the points in Golda's OCD story are far less tangible and lack the same contextual relevance.

Next try this exercise with your own OCD stories by putting yourself in someone else's shoes. Write down the concrete evidence (that comes through the five senses) or common sense they would need to be convinced that your obsessional fear is true. Another way to think about this exercise is to consider what it would take to sway a judge and jury to believe in the validity of your obsessions. Then try to recognize the ways this evidence differs from the reasoning of your OCD story.

THE PERCEPTION FLIP

This strategy encourages you to examine the role your imagination plays in generating obsessions. Take a situation that *doesn't* trigger obsessions for you—a scenario you consider safe—and try to make it into an

OCD trigger by crafting a background narrative. For example, let's say you're not particularly worried about taking a bath or shower. But what if you focus on the possibility that you could slip, fall, and break a bone; get burned by hot water; and of course, potentially drown in the bathtub? Additional risks include electric shocks; exposure to mold; bacterial and fungal infections; and chemical irritants in the soap, shampoo, or other hygiene products.

Try this exercise with different situations you generally deem safe—eating at a restaurant, visiting a doctor's office, attending public events, using household appliances—and note how creating an OCD backstory alters your thoughts and feelings. While the objective reality of the situation remains the same, your subjective experience changes (see what happens the next time you hop in the shower!). Also, notice how much you must use your imagination to generate an OCD story for something that your senses tell you is safe.

It's the same process when you construct OCD stories about situations that *do* provoke your obsessions. Can you identify the point where actual facts give way to imagined ones in relation to your obsessive fears? By consciously creating an OCD backstory for these "safe" scenarios, you can gain a deeper understanding of how your own mind amplifies harmless situations into anxiety-provoking obsessions. This awareness can help you identify the moments where reality blends into imagination in your obsessions.

BREAKING FREE FROM THE POSSIBILITY TRAP

But even if the direct evidence suggests that your obsession isn't *likely* to be true, isn't it still *possible*? Of course it is—after all, *anything* is possible. And that's exactly why possibility is not a valid reason for buying into your obsessional doubt. If you've got the kind of concrete evidence or reasoning we discussed in the previous section, you don't need to rely on possibility as a reason for buying into your obsessions. Consider the following situations:

- It's possible you won't be invited to your best friend's New Year's party, but you don't worry about it when you're holding an invitation in your hand. You trust your senses: Your common sense tells you your best friend wouldn't leave you out, and you see the invitation in your hand.

- It's possible for your luggage to get lost during a flight, but you don't worry about it once you see it on the baggage carousel. You trust your senses: You see your suitcase, and common sense tells you it's safely arrived.

- It's possible that your aunt from across the country will show up unannounced at your doorstep. But you don't worry about it because you trust your common sense that it's a long way for her to travel without checking with you first.

- It's possible a meteorite will strike your house (as happened in Alabama in 1954), but you don't worry about it because common sense tells you the odds are exceedingly low (roughly one in five million).

Now reflect on your OCD story and remember that mere possibility isn't sufficient evidence to heed. Try to identify solid evidence, from either your sensory experience or common sense, to fill in the gaps. Can you come up with any? Golda tried this exercise but couldn't identify any specific data or common sense to support her obsessional fear. What does it say about your story if you're not able to identify any evidence either?

THE LIFE SAVINGS WAGER

Another strategy to help you go beyond mere possibility as a reason for accepting your obsessional thoughts and doubts is called the life savings wager. Here's how it works: The next time you're face-to-face with an obsession, picture yourself having to stake your life savings on its validity. If you bet incorrectly, you'll lose all the money you've saved up, leaving you penniless. While you don't have to be 100% sure of your choice (it's a *wager,* after all), you do have to place the bet one way or the other. Would you bet on the obsession being valid?

This hypothetical bet forces you to look beyond mere possibility and weigh other forms of evidence to gauge the legitimacy of your obsession. You might be surprised to hear that in my professional experience working with individuals with OCD, everyone always makes the "correct" guess, indicating their ability to consider solid, credible evidence.

When I used this technique with Golda, she confidently bet that her obsession was invalid and that she would never kill Ben. When I asked her *why* she would bet against her obsession, she pointed out that she wasn't a violent person and that her love for Ben meant she would never harm him. We then examined the difference between *these* reasons and the justifications she was using to support her OCD story. You can try the same technique: Write down the reasons you would bet against the legitimacy of your own obsession, and think about how these reasons differ from the reasoning processes in your OCD story.

I hope you'll use the toolkit provided in this chapter in those moments when obsessions surface and threaten to interfere with daily activities. By equipping yourself with a range of coping strategies, and routinely practicing their use, you're better prepared to face the challenges that come your way and live a more fulfilling and less burdened life. However, obsessions are only one component of the OCD experience. Chapter 4 equips you with tactics to handle the compulsive urges and ritualistic behaviors that accompany obsessions.

Practical Steps for Living Well:
Quieting Obsessional Fears and Doubts

Shift your perspective on obsessional thoughts:

- Remember that everyone experiences intrusive unwanted thoughts.
- Know that these thoughts are part of your vivid imagination and not facts.

Change your relationship with obsessions:

- Take obsessions "along for the ride" by jotting them down and keeping them with you.

Discredit your obsessions:

- Look for the flawed logic that underlies your beliefs in your obsessions.
- Compare the flawed logic with concrete evidence and common sense.
- Ask yourself whether you would bet your life savings on the validity of your obsessions.

4

riding out
compulsive urges

If you're grappling with OCD symptoms—whether you're receiving treatment or not, and even if you've had successful treatment—you're prone to urges to perform compulsive rituals that can interfere with your daily routine. But these urges don't have to push you around and lead you to get stuck doing rituals. This chapter offers a set of strategies for sailing though and riding out these compulsive urges without succumbing to them. A necessary starting point is to become fully aware of the timing and patterns of your rituals so that you're ready for "high- risk" situations and can be proactive in getting prepared to use the strategies in this chapter. The strategies themselves involve different methods of delaying and modifying rituals and carrying out competing responses to disrupt them. You'll learn how to cultivate healthy support from family and friends that will help with your efforts to manage compulsive urges. Finally, I'll show you how to reward yourself for abstaining from rituals. Armed with these strategies, you'll be well on your way to a life less encumbered by OCD's demands.

Taking Notice of Your Rituals

The first step in riding out compulsive urges and reducing rituals is gaining awareness of the times when you're prone to engaging in these behavior patterns. Whether it's certain situations, specific obsessional thoughts, a particular time of day, or emotional states like anxiety or imperfection, understanding what provokes your rituals allows you to anticipate when you're likely to carry them out. And that's crucial because the effectiveness of the strategies in this chapter relies heavily on your proactive preparation. It's easy to be caught off guard since rituals can become so ingrained that you perform them automatically, almost without conscious thought. Heightening self-awareness allows you to catch these behaviors in real time, giving you the opportunity to interrupt them before they take shape. The best way to gain awareness of your ritual patterns is to keep a Ritual Awareness Log.

Your Ritual Awareness Log

Keeping a log of your rituals means taking note of when you perform these behaviors, along with basic information about the circumstances when the ritual occurred. All you really need is a notebook and pen or a way of digitally recording rituals (such as using a spreadsheet or smartphone application that allows you to take notes). But instead of journaling freehand, you'll want to give your log some structure and organization so it's easier to put the information you collect to good use. Ali's form, shown on the facing page, is a good example. Ali had obsessional doubts about mistakenly hitting pedestrians with his car.

As you can see, Ali decided to keep track of three rituals—asking for assurance, checking police websites, and checking the road. These were not only Ali's most frequent and time-consuming rituals, but also the ones that interfered most with his daily life. Can you think of the rituals that cause you the same types of difficulties in *your* life? Ali then created columns to log the date and time when he performed each ritual, as well as the situation or obsessional thought that provoked each

ALI'S RITUAL AWARENESS LOG

Ritual A: Asking for reassurance

Ritual B: Checking police websites for accident reports

Ritual C: Checking the road for accidents or injured people

Date	Time	Brief description of the situation or thought that led to the ritual	Which ritual?	Time spent
June 11	9:30 p.m.	TV news mentioned a car accident. What if I caused it when driving home today?	A	5 minutes
June 11	10:50 p.m.	In bed. Still thinking that I could have caused an accident today.	B	45 minutes
June 12	8:45 a.m.	Drove past someone walking on the side of the road. I could have hit them by mistake.	C	30 minutes
June 12	10:30 a.m.	Downtime at work. Thinking about driving past the pedestrian.	A	5 minutes
June 12	1:00 p.m.	Downtime at work. Still thinking about that pedestrian. What if I hit them?	A	5 minutes

one. To keep things simple, he assigned each of the rituals a letter so he didn't have to describe the ritual each time it occurred. Finally, he kept track of the amount of time each ritual took.

Notice that several of Ali's rituals seem to occur during downtimes—whether in bed or at work. Ali hadn't thought about this pattern before, but now he knows when he should be prepared to implement strategies for resisting compulsive urges. Not only that, seeing the amount of time he spent doing rituals each day—especially checking for accidents on websites and on the roadside—was a potent motivator for working hard to make changes.

Decide on which of *your* rituals occupies the most time, comes up most frequently, or gets in the way of living your best life. These will be the best ones to keep track of. Then think about what other information would be helpful to gather to understand how these rituals occur in patterns: Where and when do they happen? What is your emotional state (such as your anxiety level, rated on a scale from 1 to 10)? Are you alone or with other people when you carry them out? Set up your log so that it helps you become more aware of the factors that lead to your rituals. Finally, decide on a time frame for keeping track. Depending on how frequently you perform the rituals you're logging, the time frame could range from a single day to a few days or perhaps a week or more. Some people decide to keep their logs indefinitely.

Now you're ready. Whenever you perform a ritual, *promptly* record the incident in your log. Promptness is important because the longer you wait, the easier it is to forget important details. And the more accurate your log, the more it will help you. Take time to routinely go over and reflect on what you've written down (perhaps at the end of each day). Try to identify patterns: Are there consistent triggers? Do you find particular times of the day more challenging than others? Use the insights from your log to develop a strategy for addressing these rituals once you've read the rest of this chapter.

Keeping a log of your own behavior can be a demanding process. Here are a few more things to keep in mind as you track your rituals:

- Sharing your log with someone you trust can provide added layers of accountability and perspective.
- If real-time journaling seems tedious, you can set periodic reminders on your phone to pause and record your rituals.
- Keep your log with you as much as possible so you can quickly and accurately record your rituals in real time.
- You might also feel uncomfortable when confronting the reality of how much you ritualize.

Despite these obstacles, logging rituals gets easier with time as it becomes part of your routine. So stick with it, even if it seems tedious at first. You might also find that the very act of keeping track helps you reduce your rituals. When you approach this exercise with determination, it becomes a potent tool for self-awareness and behavior change that you can use in deploying the following strategies.

Delaying Your Rituals

Living with OCD is like being caught in a relentless tidal wave of intrusive thoughts and urges to do rituals. But what if, instead of being overwhelmed by these waves, you could learn to ride them out gracefully? Here are some strategies to help you delay the pull of your OCD rituals, allowing the urge to pass without acting on it.

Postponing Rituals

One strategy for managing compulsive urges is to intentionally postpone the ritual. Even if it's just for a brief moment, like a minute or two; or, if possible, for hours or days. Each moment of resistance helps you get stronger in the face of anxiety and the compulsive urge. For instance, when faced with an urge to engage in ritualistic behaviors like repeating prayers, seeking reassurance, washing, cleaning, or checking, challenge yourself to put the ritual off for five minutes. After this period, try to extend your resistance for another 5—or maybe 10—minutes. Continue this pattern, pushing yourself to longer and longer intervals. You'll see that in time, if you don't give in, you gain more self-confidence and the urge to ritualize eventually passes.

One evening Ali found himself obsessing over whether he might have inadvertently caused a car accident without realizing it. Typically this obsession would immediately lead him to scour the internet for any evidence he could find related to this imagined mishap. Recognizing this behavior as a ritual, he chose to postpone it by half an hour and watch a show instead. After the initial 30 minutes, he was still obsessing, so he planned for another 30-minute delay. Eventually he became engrossed in another episode of his show and forgot all about the obsession and compulsion.

When you're in the process of delaying a ritual, focus on continuing with your daily tasks or indulge in a pleasant activity you'd usually avoid during heightened anxiety. While refocusing on something else is challenging, it reaffirms that obsessions don't have to bully you and dictate your actions. Postponing rituals not only offers relief from immediate compulsions but also provides an opportunity to apply the coping mechanisms for quieting obsessive thoughts that you learned in Chapter 3.

Go Surfing!

A useful metaphor is to think of compulsive urges as waves at the beach. Just like when you're at the ocean, your urges to do rituals roll in, rise, reach a peak, crest, and then eventually subside. So you can literally think of yourself "riding them out" or "surfing on them" until they have crested and diminished. This concept is grounded in ACT, and it helps you *experience* the drive to perform rituals without any immediate reaction. Remember in Chapter 3 that a useful strategy for quieting obsessions is to give them a label? You can use the same trick with compulsive urges. For instance, when Ali felt the urge to perform a checking ritual, he would tell himself something like "I can feel the urge to drive back and check the road. It's rolling in like a wave toward the shore. But instead of being overcome by it, I'm going to get out my surfboard, catch it, and surf on it until it passes." Notice that Ali visualized himself being in *contact* with the urge, but not being consumed by it. By acknowledging these urges and allowing them to ebb and flow without giving in to them, you can reduce their hold on you, which gradually breaks the cycle of OCD.

Here's an exercise to try either when you have an urge to perform a ritual or when you're in a situation that is likely to provoke a ritual: Find a comfortable and quiet spot. Close your eyes and visualize a beach with waves rolling in. Each wave represents an urge or compulsion. Let yourself feel the urge building up like a rising wave. Remind yourself, "This is just an urge, and like a wave, it will pass. I can surf on it until it does." Let yourself feel the urge to ritualize, *but you're riding on it—not giving in to it.* Stick with the visualization for 5–10 minutes, then take a moment to acknowledge the strength it took to feel these urges without reacting. When you practice this exercise routinely, it builds resilience and self-awareness, allowing you to navigate your compulsions with a newfound sense of control.

Modifying Your Rituals

If you're having trouble putting off your rituals, or if you're not ready to stop completely at this point, the next best thing is to do the ritual in "the wrong way." That is, change some aspect of the behavior so that you're doing it "incorrectly." For instance, if you follow an orderly checking routine, you could change the order in which you compulsively check the locks, doors, and appliances. If you have strict shower rituals, you could practice washing your body parts the "wrong" way (perhaps in reverse order or for a shorter amount of time). If counting is part of your rituals, you could change the number you count to or even count incorrectly (for example, 1, 4, 2, 8, 5) so that you lose track. The object is to purposely feel like you didn't do the ritual well enough—like you have unfinished business and need to go back and do it over again. *But don't!* If you can allow yourself to feel like you've ritualized "incompletely," you're one step closer to not needing the ritual at all.

This strategy is especially helpful if you have rituals that need to be carried out "perfectly" or according to certain "rules." Lauren had invented her own strict guidelines for her hand-washing rituals. She believed she needed to wash this way to get her hands "perfectly clean" and avoid contamination: First she washed the front and back of both hands for one minute; then she washed between her fingers for 30 seconds; then up to a certain point on her wrists, and so on. Using this exercise, she first stopped using a timer during her washing. Then she modified her routine by rinsing the palms of her hands only once, and she completely refrained from washing between her fingers. This modification made Lauren feel like the ritual wasn't "good enough," which was the goal.

Almost any compulsive ritual that you carry out according to a set of rules can be revamped. You can also use ritual modification with subtle or very brief rituals. Ali would often quickly check the rear-view mirror to make sure he hadn't hit anyone with his car, so he put a piece of tape on the mirror to partially obstruct his view when he engaged in this kind of checking. If you check doors and on/off switches just by looking at them, you could try doing this ritual in dim light. You can also change up your mental compulsions. If you have prayer rituals, for example, you can say the prayer incorrectly. If you feel you have to repeat certain "safe" or "lucky" words or phrases, you can do so in a different language or by visualizing the words being misspelled—anything that makes you feel like the ritual is foiled. If you have reviewing rituals, purposely remember what happened *incorrectly*.

Revamping Your Rituals

To use this strategy, start by planning out exactly how you're going to change up each particular ritual that you've been keeping track of. Grab a pen and paper and write down parameters such as (1) the details of how you perform the ritual (such as the order of individual behaviors like Lauren's hand washing), (2) how many times you engage in the behavior or how long it lasts, (3) where you perform the ritual, and (4) the role of anyone else involved. Then think about what you can do differently and write down these new parameters. It's not necessary to make changes to *every* aspect of the ritual—although the more you alter, the better. The important factor is modifying the ritual in a way that makes it feel incomplete. When you consistently practice carrying out the ritual incorrectly or incompletely, the urge to carry it out will gradually decrease.

Using Competing Responses

Another strategy for riding out compulsive urges is to perform an alternative behavior instead—which I call a *competing response*. One approach is to use a competing response that's physically incompatible with doing the ritual. For instance, if you have a compulsion to repeatedly unlock and lock the door, you could hold an object in each hand

and walk away from the door until the urge to check passes. Another method is to simply distract yourself from the urge by engaging in a more pleasant or otherwise constructive behavior, such as a hobby or exercise. By consistently practicing these types of competing responses, you disrupt the OCD cycle and redirect your brain's neural pathways, gradually lessening the automatic nature of the ritual.

Using "Anti-Rituals"

Anti-rituals are activities that either prevent or significantly hinder your ability to perform a ritual. It's helpful to arm yourself with a variety of anti-rituals for when those compelling urges strike. So dedicate some time to brainstorming activities that directly conflict with your rituals. Here are some ideas to inspire you.

For checking rituals:

- Remove yourself from where the checking would occur.
- Turn off the lights so it's more difficult to see what you're checking.
- Cover what you're checking with a piece of paper so you can't see the position of the switch or dial.

For hand-washing rituals:

- Put on a pair of gloves.
- Apply hand lotion.
- Engage in an activity that requires both hands, like holding a book.
- Make sure you're as far as possible from sinks.
- Have someone hide the hand sanitizer (or better yet, just throw it out or avoid buying it).

For aligning or arranging rituals:

- Deliberately rearrange things in a different order and then immediately engage in a distracting activity, like calling a friend or listening to music.

For reassurance-seeking rituals:

- Instruct anyone you ask for assurance to give you the "wrong" answer (later in this chapter I'll cover more strategies for getting help from other people).
- Stay away from people you ask for reassurance (when applicable).
- Disconnect the computer from the internet when the urge to search online arises.

Next, plan how long you'll stick with the anti-ritual. You might try it for a specific amount of time—perhaps longer than you think you *could*—to prove to yourself that you're able to manage the compulsive urge. Another strategy is to engage in and stick with the anti-ritual behavior until the compulsive urge fades. It ensures that your brain acknowledges this new behavior as an alternative to the ritual.

One key to successfully counteracting rituals is using the anti-ritual immediately upon sensing the compulsive urge. Doing so establishes a strong link between the compulsion and its counteraction. Consistency is also critical. The more routinely you use the competing anti-ritual response, the more it becomes solidified as a pattern, diminishing the urge to complete the OCD ritual and paving the way for living with more freedom of choice. Finally, after engaging in the competing behavior, rate its effectiveness on a scale of 1 to 10. This will help you identify which anti-ritual strategies are most beneficial for you.

Using Distraction

The concept behind distracting yourself when compulsive urges show up is simple: By engaging in another activity, you leave less mental bandwidth available for intrusive thoughts or the urges to act on them. The best distractions are activities that both divert your attention and also contribute to your well-being, like stretching and exercising. Physical activity releases endorphins, which can help in elevating your mood and self-confidence. Creative activities like drawing, painting, or playing a musical instrument can be equally potent in pulling your attention away from the compulsive urge, as can reading, listening to a podcast, cooking (savoring the tastes and smells), or even a warm bath.

Begin by listing activities you enjoy or would like to explore. Over the next week, whenever you're in a situation likely to trigger a compulsive urge—or you feel one beginning to rise—try out an activity from your list. Remember that not every distraction will work every time, so it's about finding what fits best for each situation. Also, don't just sit there watching the clock, hoping that your compulsive urge will subside as quickly as possible. Focusing on the time while you white-knuckle through the experience will only prolong the process and prevent you from rewiring those all-important neural pathways. Instead, try mindfully throwing yourself into your distraction. Don't be surprised if you occasionally need to change up your repertoire of distractions as your preferences for different kinds of activities change. Finally, as with the anti-ritual behaviors, keep track of how well the different distraction tactics worked for you.

Getting Support from Family and Friends

Do family members or friends pitch in to help with your rituals? Maybe someone wipes down the mail and groceries before bringing them into the house because of your contamination fear. Perhaps someone cuts your food for you because you're afraid of knives. Does your religious or spiritual leader listen to excessive confessions or give you reassurance that you haven't sinned? Do your parents send you money to buy heavy-duty cleaning supplies and extra toilet paper (or perhaps they buy these items for you)?

It might seem like a loving gesture when someone else goes out of their way to help with your rituals or avoidance. And in the moment, it might even reduce your obsessional thinking and anxiety. But the reality is that this kind of "help" won't do you any favors when it comes to managing compulsive urges and living well in the long run. For one thing, regardless of who is doing them, rituals reinforce your obsessional fears and strengthen the OCD cycle. Another problem is that when others help with rituals and avoidance on your behalf, it can lead to an unhealthy reliance on them to manage your anxiety for you. Over time this kind of dependence escalates the number and complexity of your rituals, making you rely on these other people more and more. And while friends and family might be willing to participate in the short term, as rituals expand or become more frequent, they put a strain on relationships. All of these points mean that to enjoy a more fulfilling life, you'll need to guide your friends and family to help you in healthier ways to ride out compulsive urges. Here's how to proceed.

GUIDING YOUR LOVED ONES

Make a list of (1) the ways that people in your life participate in your rituals and (2) the changes they can make—either stopping their participation or helping you use the techniques described earlier in this chapter. Then organize a meeting with your loved ones and offer clear guidance on what you would like them to do (or *not* do) from now on. For example, explain that you would like them to refuse if you request their help with a ritual. Ali called a family meeting to discuss how he was going to work on reducing his reassurance seeking. He then asked his family to respond to any questions about car accidents by saying encouraging things like "Remember you wanted me not to answer those kinds of questions anymore. I know this is tough for you, but I also know that you're strong and you can get through this without my reassurance."

Ali also came up with the idea of sending his friends and family a letter that explained the OCD vicious cycle and how he would like their help getting *through* compulsive urges *without doing rituals*. Here's what he wrote—consider something similar for your inner circle.

> *Dear Family and Friends,*
>
> *I'm taking steps to reduce how OCD impacts my life, and I hope you can help me. It won't require much work on your part; actually, it will mean doing **less!***
>
> *I will be trying some new strategies to help me resist the urge to ask you for reassurance, but if I slip up and ask anyway, I would like you to remind me of the following instead of giving me reassurance:*
>
> - *It looks like you're having obsessional doubts. How can I help you use one of the new strategies you're practicing?*
> - *Remember you sent me a letter saying I shouldn't answer these*

*kinds of questions anymore? I'm going to honor your request because
I love you, and I know you can manage the anxiety using your new
strategies.*

*When you say these things, there's a possibility that I will try even
harder to get you to participate in my rituals. If I do, please don't give in. I
might seem very upset and anxious, but the obsessions and anxiety are not
harmful. Instead, please encourage me to use the new skills I'm practicing
to quiet obsessions and ride out compulsive urges.*

*I'm grateful for your support and encouragement as I go through this
learning process. I don't want OCD to get in the way of our family/friend-
ship any longer.*

With love,
Ali

Positive Reinforcement

Positive reinforcement involves providing a favorable incentive—
a reward—following a desired behavior. This strategy bolsters the
recurrence of the desired behavior by linking it with positive results.
Essentially, when you're rewarded for a particular action, you're more
inclined to repeat it in the future. For people with OCD, this approach
can be instrumental in reducing rituals. Rewarding yourself for successfully managing compulsive urges without giving in heightens
your chances of repeated success. Used effectively, rewards shift your
mind-set: Instead of focusing on the distress of obsessive thoughts, you
think about the upcoming reward. The prospect of a reward becomes a
potent driving force, especially when the compulsion to engage in rituals feels overpowering. Rewards also lift your self-esteem, reinforcing
your confidence in managing rituals. Furthermore they cultivate self-
awareness because you become more observant of your own behavior
and the emotions and situations that induce them. You can see the
value in establishing your own reward system to promote resistance
to compulsive urges. Recommendations for how to achieve effective
incentives are detailed in the following section.

Rewarding Yourself for Riding Out Compulsive Urges

DEFINE CLEAR CRITERIA

Begin with deciding on what qualifies as successfully riding out a compulsive urge or resisting a ritual. Is it resisting one time? Multiple times in a day? Setting clear goals will help you determine when a reward has been earned.

CHOOSE YOUR REWARDS

Next, select the rewards you'll give yourself when you meet your goals. Opt for rewards that genuinely spark your joy or satisfaction. The more personal and meaningful they are, the more they'll motivate you to work hard. Additionally, make sure to scale your rewards so they match the size of the goals reached: Save higher-value or more special rewards for moments of more remarkable resistance or when you've achieved a more substantial goal. Here are some examples of rewards you might choose:

- Buy something for your hobby.
- Enjoy a nice meal at a fancy restaurant.
- See a movie.
- Go for a spa treatment or massage.
- Attend a show or concert you've been wanting to see.
- Pay someone to do the yard work or housecleaning this week.
- Find some time to be by yourself.
- Take a weekend getaway.

STAY ACCOUNTABLE

Make sure to reward yourself only when you've earned it! Cutting corners and giving yourself rewards that haven't been genuinely earned weakens the effectiveness of the reward. On the other hand, when you adhere to your reward criteria, you build trust in yourself, which is foundational to resisting rituals. To this end, share your plan and progress with trusted relatives or friends. Your loved ones can encourage you, celebrate with you, and help hold you accountable.

DOCUMENT AND REEVALUATE

Documenting your progress using a journal allows you to track how you're doing, savor your victories, and review challenges. Finally, evaluate and adjust your plan on a regular basis. As your circumstances or challenges evolve, your strategy might need tweaking to remain effective. Remember, the goal is consistent progress rather than perfection. Rewards are a testament to each step forward that you take, celebrating growth and resilience.

Navigating the labyrinth of OCD and its compulsive urges is a journey, but with the right strategies you can reclaim the reins of your daily life. As I've emphasized, recognition of compulsive urges, preparation, and consistency in using the strategies in this chapter are the linchpins of success. Understanding these strategies is a great start, but it's the consistent, methodical use of them that will help you manage compulsive urges without giving in. Remember, success with these tactics takes time, patience, and practice. As you continue your path toward a life less dictated by compulsive urges, I encourage you to refine and personalize these techniques. Adapt them to resonate with your experiences and challenges. Seek joy in the rewards you give yourself, celebrating each moment of resistance as a victory over OCD. While OCD might be a part of your life, it doesn't define who you are. Armed with knowledge, bolstered by consistent effort, and supported by loved ones, you are more than equipped to chart a path toward a fulfilling life where compulsive rituals no longer hold sway! The next chapter focuses on time management and organizational skills, which are valuable tools for reducing OCD triggers and improving your overall quality of life.

Practical Steps for Living Well:
Riding Out Compulsive Urges

Track your rituals:

- Use a notebook, spreadsheet, or smartphone app to log your rituals.
- List how others participate in your rituals.
- Review your log regularly to identify patterns and triggers.

Delay your rituals:

- Start with a few minutes and gradually work up to a longer delay.
- Visualize the urge as a wave you can ride while you do a routine task or enjoyable activity.

Modify your compulsions:

- Change the order, duration, or manner of the ritual.
- Embrace the feeling that the ritual is incomplete.

Use competing responses:

- Perform an alternative behavior that hinders your ability to perform a ritual.
- Distract yourself with hobbies, exercise, or other enjoyable activities.

Maintain consistency with rewards and support:

- Reward yourself for delaying or abstaining from compulsive behaviors.
- Let your family and friends know how they can support you as you reduce your rituals.

5

taking control
of your time

Being able to manage time effectively is crucial for just about everyone. If you're living with OCD, it's especially vital because of the particular ways obsessions and compulsions affect your daily life. But it's about finding a balance—structuring your time to manage OCD effectively while also being flexible and self-compassionate when OCD-related interruptions occur. On the one hand, by mastering the art of organization and establishing a structured routine, you create a framework that can help you stay focused on important tasks, enhancing your efficiency and reducing the time available for obsessions and compulsions to creep in. On the other hand, the very nature of OCD means that intrusive thoughts and compulsive urges can still disrupt the most well-planned schedules. Even if you've been making progress on reducing your rituals, the ones you still perform can be time-consuming and interfere with completing routine tasks. Acknowledging that these realities coexist is key, and a balanced approach can help in some important ways:

- Establishing a structured routine reduces the time you lose to compulsions.
- Effective time management leads to less rushing, reduced stress, and fewer triggers for OCD symptoms.

- Achieving tasks on time and meeting goals improves your sense of self-worth.

- You'll be better able to carve out adequate time for practicing the strategies in this book (or in therapy) to help with managing OCD.

So in the spirit of this chapter, let's dive right in without another moment's delay!

Prioritizing Tasks to Minimize OCD's Influence

Organizing your day when you're living with OCD is a challenge. But even if obsessions and compulsions are present, *prioritizing* is a strategy you can use to create structure and provide a foundation for the other strategies you'll learn in this chapter. When you have a clear road map steering you toward what's essential and requires immediate attention in your life, you can lessen the paralysis that arises from OCD. By addressing crucial tasks first, you'll ensure that significant responsibilities are taken care of and cultivate a rewarding sense of accomplishment. Prioritizing also sharpens your ability to make decisions, fostering adaptability in the face of OCD and its unexpected challenges. Here are some strategies to help you do so.

Important versus *Urgent* Activities

Our activities can be productive in two ways: They can be *important* and they can be *urgent*. A task is *important* to the extent that it contributes significantly to your personal or professional life—your health and relationships, work or school, and other things that you value. In other words, important tasks get you closer to the core values you identified in Chapter 2. Examples might include planning a major project at work that could propel your career forward, setting aside time for exercise or other self-care activities that enhance your well-being, and volunteering at the food bank to serve those in need. Consider your core values, and then identify *your* tasks and activities of importance.

Urgent tasks, on the other hand, are activities that require immediate attention for one reason or another. Not addressing them promptly could lead to negative consequences. You'd want to drop what you're doing if you had an overflowing toilet, got an email from a teacher or boss requiring immediate clarification, or received a phone call from a close friend or relative in crisis who needs help right now. Urgent tasks often—but not always—arise suddenly and unexpectedly; and although they don't always align with your core values and long-term goals, they're time sensitive and can't be postponed.

You're probably wondering where compulsive rituals fit within this framework. They might seem *important* because their goal is often to prevent the disastrous consequences you fear. But they also might seem *urgent* because you experience pressure to complete them as soon as possible. Of course, as we've seen, the reality is that rituals are neither important nor urgent. It's just that OCD has a way of making it seem like the sky is falling when obsessional fears are really just false alarms.

The Activity Log

How much time do you spend on important versus urgent tasks? How much time is unproductive or consumed by OCD? If you're like most people with OCD, you probably underestimate how much time you spend on compulsive rituals and avoidance behaviors. Getting a better handle on how you spend your day will help you set priorities and increase your time spent on important matters.

I suggest using the Activity Log on page 70 to monitor your daily actions. Although it's similar to the Ritual Awareness Log in Chapter 4, it's more comprehensive and allows you to track activities in addition to compulsive rituals. It also helps you see your OCD behaviors in context with other activities. Here are some suggestions for how to fill out the Activity Log.

- Fill it out in "real time" throughout the day, rather than waiting until the end of the day, when you're tired and likely to forget or underestimate key activities. You might need to take the log with you if you leave home so you'll have it handy throughout the day. Make sure you record *everything* you spend more than

ACTIVITY LOG

Time	Activity	Remarks	Category
			I U W OCD
			I U W OCD
			I U W OCD
			I U W OCD
			I U W OCD
			I U W OCD
			I U W OCD
			I U W OCD
			I U W OCD
			I U W OCD
			I U W OCD
			I U W OCD
			I U W OCD
			I U W OCD
			I U W OCD
			I U W OCD
			I U W OCD
			I U W OCD

a few minutes doing. If it's more convenient, create your own electronic version of the log that you can use on a phone or tablet.

- In the far-left column, note the time of day when you started and finished the activity. Try to be precise—use a clock or watch.

- There's no need to be overly detailed; just use terms that will allow you to recognize the activity upon reviewing the log: emailing, meeting, answering phone calls, socializing, driving, getting a haircut, eating, driving, shopping, practicing a sport or musical instrument, surfing the web, exercising, watching TV, napping, cleaning, checking, mentally ritualizing, and so on.

- If you have any comments about doing the activity, enter them in the "Remarks" column.

- Don't do anything with the "Category" column just yet; we'll get to this column in the next section.

- Make copies of the blank form for future use and log your activities for at least three "typical" days.

LEARNING FROM YOUR LOG

Once you have some information about how you're spending your time, you can analyze it and find out how much your daily activities match up with your values:

1. Identify those activities that are in line with your values and goals, that is, those that are *important*. For each one, circle *I* in the "Category" column.

2. Identify activities that you did because they were *urgent*. Maybe there was external pressure making you feel like you had to get this activity done. In the "Category" column. circle *U* for each of these activities.

3. For any activity that represents a waste of your time—it doesn't accomplish anything important or urgent—circle *W*.

4. Circle *OCD* for any activities related to obsessions, compulsive rituals, and avoidance.

Everyone wastes some of their time each day doing things that are neither important nor urgent, so don't beat yourself up over that. And if you have OCD, some of that wasted time will be spent on avoidance or rituals. Still, if you're looking for ways to manage your time better, these are the categories to minimize. Look back at the strategies for resisting compulsive rituals in Chapter 4. Here's where you can really put them to good use. Examine other sources of wasted time, and think about what you could do to reduce or eliminate them as well. In the same vein, increasing your time spent on activities related to important goals and values will help make you more productive.

But go slowly—don't try to make too many changes at once or you risk feeling overwhelmed and scrapping your plans altogether. Instead, alter your routine a bit at a time—perhaps adding one new change each week. Over time the changes will add up, and you'll find yourself being more productive and satisfied. You might again put pen to paper and create an action plan for reducing wasteful and OCD-related activities. Specify which ideas from Chapter 4 you'll try out each week for the next several weeks.

The ABCD Method

If you're feeling overwhelmed by the number of things you've got to get done, the ABCD method is a strategy for prioritizing these activities. It can help you increase productivity and efficiency and reduce the impact of OCD by ensuring that your most critical tasks are completed first. It's an easy concept to grasp and put into action. I've broken it down/conceptualized it into these steps that you can follow:

CATEGORIZE YOUR UPCOMING TASKS

What do you need to get done in the near future? Start by making a list and assigning each task the letter A, B, C, or D to represent one of the following categories:

• **A-tasks (important and urgent):** These tasks need to be the highest priority. If not done immediately, there could be significant costs. Some examples include completing a project for work or school that is due tomorrow and could have a major impact on your overall performance, attending a scheduled therapy appointment, taking prescribed medication on time, or sending an important email that you've been obsessing over for correctness.

- **B-tasks (important but not urgent):** These tasks contribute to your long-term goals but don't need immediate attention. Good examples include activities that support your well-being and your values, but aren't time sensitive, such as exercising or reading a book to enhance your professional knowledge. Tasks you might do to make OCD more manageable also fit into this category, such as organizing your living space to reduce OCD triggers and planning a relaxing activity for the weekend.

- **C-tasks (urgent but not necessarily important):** This category includes tasks that need quick attention but may not directly impact your well-being or significantly contribute to your goals in life. They're often distractions that may unexpectedly demand your time, such as dealing with an unknown charge on your credit card.

- **D-tasks (neither important nor urgent):** D-tasks might be enjoyable or routine but aren't pressing. They're low priority and could even be eliminated from your to-do list. Examples include browsing social media, shopping online, or reorganizing your desk.

START WITH A-TASKS

Begin by taking care of those that are both urgent and important so you can reduce potential anxiety or stress triggers. For instance, if you've had obsessions over sending a certain email, drafting and sending it as an A-task can provide relief. Next, move on to B-tasks, C-tasks, and finally D-tasks.

USE TOOLS AND REMINDERS

Living with OCD might mean that sometimes tasks feel overwhelming or are overshadowed by compulsions. Set reminders or alarms, especially for A-tasks, to ensure they don't get overlooked. This can be particularly helpful if doing compulsive rituals leads to forgetting or avoiding certain tasks.

REASSESS REGULARLY

Your priorities may shift, especially on days when OCD symptoms are stronger. It's okay to reassess and rearrange tasks based on how you feel. It's helpful to get into the habit of continually categorizing tasks that come your way so that you don't fall behind.

BE SELF-COMPASSIONATE

It's okay if you don't get to every task on your list. Celebrate what you do achieve and understand that living with OCD means that some days might be more challenging than others. Understand that by incorporating the ABCD method you're streamlining your day, offering clarity, and reducing potential sources of anxiety.

Structuring Your Day to Minimize OCD's Interference

Adding structure helps us all navigate our days more efficiently, but living with OCD can make planning even the most routine day seem overwhelming. Maybe certain activities trigger obsessional fears and lead to getting stuck doing rituals. Perhaps the unpredictability of some situations provokes anxiety and avoidance. Along with the ABCD method, I recommend using a planner or digital calendar to organize your day—if you don't already do so. Include specific time blocks for activities, chores, work or school, and relaxation. Here again you'll also need to be realistic about how much time OCD symptoms might take up. The strategies described in this section can help you effectively plan your day.

SET UP YOUR SCHEDULE

First, decide between a paper-and-pencil planner and a digital calendar. Some people with OCD find writing in a planner satisfying or calming, while others prefer the convenience of a digital tool. An added benefit of electronic devices is that you can set reminders.

Next jot down any fixed appointments or commitments in your planner. This might include therapy sessions, work meetings, or other important obligations (A-tasks). If there are other activities or tasks that you need to get done, find a place for them in your calendar as well.

BREAK DOWN COMPLEX TASKS

When larger and more complex tasks that seem overwhelming are involved—especially those that trigger obsessions or compulsions—I suggest breaking them down into smaller steps to put on your calendar. This will give you a sense of controllability and predictability that can reduce your anxiety. For instance, if the task of organizing your room is looming over you, try thinking about it in terms of tackling smaller components such as (1) making the bed, (2) sorting the laundry, (3) clearing off the nightstand, and (4) vacuuming the floor. Then allocate a realistic time frame for each activity. Thinking about tasks this way not only makes them seem more manageable, but also allows you to decide if you want to spread them across different days or do them all at once. You'll also need to decide the order in which you want to complete the smaller steps. Maybe you'd prefer to handle the easiest tasks first to build momentum or perhaps start with the hardest ones to get them out of the way. Whatever approach you decide on, this process provides clear stopping points, allowing for breaks if OCD symptoms become intense. The predictability and structure can also serve as an antidote to the uncertainty and distress that OCD often brings.

PLAN MINDFULLY

The next step is to estimate how long each activity or task will take. Be realistic and account for any OCD-related interruptions you anticipate with each task. Since OCD can be mentally exhausting, be sure to schedule short breaks to engage in a calming activity and reset your focus. On a related note, be sure to incorporate self-care activities in your daily routine, whether it's reading, listening to music, or taking a short walk. This kind of activity serves as a mental breather, but you can also think of it as a reward for your efforts. Avoiding overscheduling is another key to managing OCD effectively because overloading your schedule can exacerbate obsessions and compulsions. Finally, setting realistic goals, prioritizing tasks, and learning to say no help you maintain a manageable schedule.

MAINTAIN FLEXIBILITY

At the end of each day, review your planner. Celebrate the tasks you completed, and consider whether there's a better way to approach the ones you didn't get to. Adjust for the next day, learning and growing from your experiences. Remember, your goal isn't perfection. It's about creating a structure that supports and respects your unique journey with OCD, making each day a bit more manageable and predictable. Consider your schedule a guideline or road map rather than a strict rulebook. It's okay if your day doesn't go exactly as planned. If you need to reschedule tasks because of an unexpected OCD flare-up, that's okay. Be gentle with yourself!

USE A TIMER

If compulsive rituals continue to interfere with getting things done, consider using a timer. The idea is to decide on a specific duration—such as five minutes—to limit your compulsive activity. First, challenge yourself to complete rituals only within that time frame, gradually reducing the time allocated as you progress. But this approach is not just about rushing through the compulsion and saving time; you can also use the timer to interrupt your rituals midstream, which will gradually retrain your brain to withstand obsessional discomfort, breaking the cycle of OCD. As you become accustomed to this practice, progressively decrease the time allotted for rituals, fostering more and more resilience and reclaiming precious minutes of your day. Keep a journal as a tangible tracker of your journey and your achievements. Celebrate every moment reclaimed from the clutches of compulsions, however small it may seem, as each victory brings you a step closer to more functionality, control, and a life less dominated by OCD.

Minimizing Distractions

Navigating through the day with OCD can often feel like a journey through a labyrinth, filled with potential distractions at every turn. The key to effective time management in this context is to minimize these distractions, creating a clear and focused environment conducive to productivity and well-being. Here are some tips and strategies to help you identify, reduce, and eliminate distractions, paving the way for a smoother, more controlled daily routine.

DETECT YOUR DIVERSIONS

To tackle distractions, you first need to identify them. Pay attention to your surroundings and note what tends to pull your focus away from the task at hand. Is it the constant pinging of notifications? The clutter on your desk? Interruptions from family members? Perhaps it's obsessional thoughts and urges to do compulsive rituals. By becoming aware of these distractions, you can start to address them proactively.

SILENCE THE PINGS!

In our hyperconnected world, digital distractions are a significant challenge. Start by turning off nonessential notifications on your phone and computer. Create specific times to check emails and social media, rather than allowing them to intrude on your focus throughout the day. Consider using website blockers or productivity apps designed to minimize digital distractions.

CREATE A "WORK SANCTUARY"

Having a designated workspace can do wonders for your concentration. Ensure this space is tidy, organized, and free from clutter. Personalize it with items that are calming and help you focus, but be mindful not to overdecorate your workspace, as clutter can become a distraction in itself. One more thing—and this is probably obvious: Try to avoid keeping items that provoke OCD symptoms in your work sanctuary. The last thing you need is to have your obsessional fears provoked when you're trying to focus on something important!

SET SOCIAL BOUNDARIES

If you live with family or roommates, clear communication is key. Set boundaries and share your schedule with them, letting them know when you need uninterrupted time. If possible, use visual cues like a closed door or even a "Do Not Disturb" sign to signal when you are in focused work mode.

SCHEDULE BLOCKS OF "FOCUSED TIME"

Establishing a routine with designated time blocks for specific activities can help minimize distractions. Use a method like the Pomodoro technique, in which you work for 25 minutes and then take a 5-minute break to create a structured work rhythm.

REFLECT AND ADJUST

At the end of each day or week, reflect on what worked and what didn't. Were there distractions you hadn't anticipated? Or perhaps a strategy that worked exceptionally well? Use these reflections to continuously adjust and refine your approach, ensuring ongoing improvement and greater control over your environment.

Minimizing distractions is an important component of effective time management when you have OCD. By proactively identifying and addressing potential disruptions, creating a designated workspace, setting clear boundaries, and establishing focused routines, you can create an environment that supports concentration, productivity, and well-being. Remember, this is a journey of continuous improvement, and each step you take toward minimizing distractions is a step toward a more focused, controlled, and fulfilling life.

Overcoming Procrastination

Let's not delay the section on procrastination any further! Indeed, OCD can involve several ingredients that lead to procrastination: anxiety, perfectionism, fears of making mistakes, indecisiveness, rituals, trouble concentrating, and avoidance of discomfort. The truth is that we procrastinate when we postpone important, high-priority (often unpleasant) tasks until "later" and instead engage in less crucial activities that may be pleasant or reduce distress. It's a common human behavior pattern, and a certain amount of procrastination is perfectly normal. However, when it's excessive, or it interferes with pursuing what you value in life, it turns into a problem that can exacerbate OCD symptoms. Maybe you avoid tasks you dislike until you find yourself pulling all-nighters to meet deadlines. Or you wait so long that your performance at work or school slumps. Or you suffer social disapproval for not meeting your commitments. Any of these consequences of procrastination raises anxiety and induces OCD symptoms. Here are some strategies you can use the next time you're tempted to put off something important.

LOOK AT THE CONSEQUENCES

Make two lists: The first is a list of all the unpleasant aspects of doing the task that you're currently putting off. In the second list, write down the consequences of putting off the task. On page 80 you can see the lists that Matthew, a teacher, made about getting started with grading a stack of his students' papers, which he'd been putting off.

With these lists in hand, Matthew then thought about the discomfort of grading his class's papers versus the consequences of putting this task off even longer—you can do this with your lists as well. He realized that the consequences of *not* grading the papers would actually be *more* unpleasant than just grading them right away. It was the lesser of two evils. And thinking about it this way motivated him to set aside the time and grade the papers then and there. Try this exercise the next time you're procrastinating. You'll probably arrive at the same conclusions and make the same decision.

Matthew: Lists for Grading Papers

Unpleasant aspects	Consequences of not grading the papers
• It will take a long time.	• I'll still have to do it at some point—the papers won't grade themselves.
• It's monotonous.	• There will be even more papers to grade soon, so my work will only pile up and make me more stressed.
• There are so many other, more interesting things I could be doing.	• My students will be upset because I have been delaying getting their papers back to them, and they want to know how they did on the assignments.
	• If a student isn't doing well, I won't know and can't help them.

LINK THE TASK TO AN ACTIVITY YOU ENJOY

Like the spoonful of sugar that helps the medicine go down, when you connect an activity you don't enjoy (the "medicine") with something you like (the "sugar"), suddenly the unlikable activity doesn't seem so bad. If, for example, you're putting off unloading the dishwasher or doing other work around the house, try linking it to something you like, such as putting on your favorite music and "rocking out" while you clean or work. If you dislike exercising or grocery shopping, get a friend to go with you to chat with, show you some new exercise moves, or help you find bargains.

REWARD YOURSELF

When all else fails, set up a reward system in which you earn points for completing the tasks you've been putting off. Make a list, and when you've earned a certain number of points, buy yourself something you like.

BREAK THE TASK DOWN

As described earlier, if the whole task or job seems overwhelming and difficult to tackle all at once, there's no harm in dividing it into smaller and more manageable ("bite-size") tasks that you can feel better about doing.

While the challenges of OCD can make time management seem daunting, with consistency and the right strategies, you can lead a balanced and fulfilling life. So now that you've got a better understanding of how you spend your time and some strategies to improve your time management, you can begin making changes. But go gradually. Trying to alter too many aspects of your routine too fast can leave you feeling overwhelmed and unable to keep up with all of your adjustments— exactly what you're trying to avoid. My suggestion is to try out one new time-management strategy per week, and once you're comfortable with it, add another new strategy each week until you feel you're making progress.

Practical Steps for Living Well:
Taking Control of Your Time

Establish a structured routine:

- Use a planner or digital calendar to create a daily schedule of your appointments, work, chores, and relaxation time.
- Divide larger tasks into smaller, manageable steps to reduce anxiety and improve focus.

Prioritize tasks to minimize OCD's influence:

- Categorize tasks according to their importance and urgency to focus on what truly matters.
- Use an Activity Log to track how you spend your time and identify areas for improvement.

Minimize distractions:

- Evaluate the consequences of procrastination versus the benefits of completing tasks promptly.
- Combine tasks you dislike with activities you enjoy to make them more bearable.

6

finding a balance between privacy and disclosure

Opening up to others about something as private as having OCD can seem daunting. Maybe you've wrestled with the idea but were concerned about crafting the right message or about how people might react to you. Indeed, finding the language to truly capture your experience or explain seemingly "odd" behaviors can be tricky, and it's the same with predicting how others might respond. But remember, the decision to share your story is a personal choice. And if you elect to tell others, doing so requires careful planning about when and how to express your truth in a way that feels right for you.

That's why it's good to have a comprehensive guide to opening up about OCD, with tools and strategies for confidently navigating these important conversations. This chapter lays out the advantages and disadvantages of sharing your story and, should you decide to do so, discusses how to select the right moment, craft a clear and relatable message, and prepare for the range of reactions you might get. I'll also help you set personal boundaries so you can balance your privacy with the desire to let others know about your lived experience. Whether you're thinking of speaking about your OCD for the first time or looking to polish your approach to these conversations, this chapter is designed to steer you through the process with clarity and confidence.

To Share or Not: What to Consider

Many people choose to keep their battles with OCD private, yet I've seen numerous others draw comfort and empowerment from speaking openly about their condition. And it's not an all-or-nothing situation—there are many degrees of disclosure, as we'll explore later in this chapter. Typically, the journey to sharing starts at a juncture filled with uncertainty. In therapy, we carefully examine the potential advantages and challenges that accompany the decision to share personal experiences with OCD. But each person's path is unique, and there is no "right" or "wrong" choice. Here are some strategies for figuring out whether sharing your experiences with OCD is the right choice for you.

Deciding If the Time Is Right

Begin by taking stock of your own thoughts and feelings toward OCD and your mind-set toward discussing it with others. How comfortable are you in talking about your personal life? If the topic of OCD comes up, how do you feel? Do you find yourself wishing others better understood what you're going through? Keep in mind that your approach to answering these kinds of questions could differ depending on your audience, for example, responding to a family member as opposed to a colleague. Here are some additional questions you might consider, your answers to which can serve as a barometer for your readiness to disclose:

- What do I hope to achieve by disclosing my OCD?
- Am I ready to handle the barrage of questions that people may have?
- Am I ready to deal with a variety of reactions, ranging from supportive to misunderstanding to potentially insensitive or dismissive?

- How might sharing OCD impact my personal and professional relationships?
- Am I ready to handle any additional stress that may come from disclosing?
- What support systems do I have in place to help me through any negative aftermath?

Thinking Through the Pros and Cons

The table on page 86 highlights the potential advantages and disadvantages of informing others about your OCD diagnosis. On the positive side, letting others know can pave the way for valuable emotional support from friends and family, creating a network of understanding and care. Speaking openly can also reduce feelings of isolation and loneliness since it connects you with others who may share your experiences or who are willing to empathize with your journey. On the other hand, others may respond with misconceptions or stigmatized views, which can be disheartening (I've included a section "Addressing Misconceptions" on how to respond to these people later in this chapter). Sharing also may stir up your own strong emotions. Additionally, while friends and family may have the best intentions, they might want to give you advice that is not particularly helpful or informed.

So, it's useful to think of communicating about OCD as a balancing act that requires careful planning and patience. Remember that the decision to share is yours alone, and it's okay to take the time you need to weigh the pros and cons, knowing that if and when you choose to open up, you do so on your own terms. By taking time to consider all the key factors, you can ensure that if you do choose to share your story, you do it in a way that supports your well-being and fosters understanding. Remember, you are not alone, and support is available whether you decide to share your experience with OCD or not.

Who, When, Where, and How?

As you consider whether to confide in others, it's important to think about who in your life will provide a supportive ear and a compassionate

Potential Pros and Cons of Opening Up about OCD

Potential pros of disclosure	Potential cons of disclosure
Increased understanding. Disclosing your condition can lead to a deeper understanding from friends, family, and colleagues, fostering empathy and support.	**Misunderstanding.** People may have a limited or skewed understanding of OCD, leading to misconceptions about your experience.
Reduced stigma. Openly discussing your OCD can help break down misconceptions and reduce the stigma associated with mental health conditions.	**Stigma.** Despite growing awareness, there's still a stigma attached to mental health issues, and you may encounter negative judgments or stereotypes.
Emotional relief. Sharing your struggles can provide a sense of relief and decrease the burden of carrying a secret.	**Privacy concerns.** Once shared, information about your OCD may no longer be private, potentially affecting personal and professional relationships.
Improved relationships. Honesty about your condition can strengthen trust and intimacy in personal relationships.	**Emotional reactions.** The disclosure might elicit emotional reactions, from discomfort to overconcern, which can be challenging to manage.
Tailored support. Once others are aware, they may offer more personalized help or accommodations, especially in educational or workplace settings.	**Boundary setting.** You might have to navigate how much to share and set boundaries to prevent conversations from becoming intrusive or harmful.
Community building. You might connect with others who have OCD, creating a community that understands and supports one another.	**Impact on relationships.** People may treat you differently, either by being overly cautious or by not providing the support you expected.
Self-acceptance. Talking about your OCD can promote self-acceptance, self-esteem, personal growth, and resilience.	**Workplace dynamics.** Sharing your OCD could impact your career or work environment in unforeseen ways.
Role modeling. By being open about your condition, you can serve as a role model to others who might be afraid to disclose their own struggles.	**Unwanted attention.** Becoming the focus of attention can be uncomfortable or lead to unwanted questions or curiosity.
Educational opportunities. You have the chance to promote a broader understanding and compassion within your community.	**Relapse concerns.** Stress from negative interactions has the potential to contribute to a relapse or worsening of symptoms.

heart upon hearing your story. Additionally, you'll want to choose an appropriate moment and environment. Finally, the method of communication—be it an in-person conversation or through digital means like texting or social media—carries its own set of advantages and drawbacks.

WHO SHOULD I TELL?

Start by identifying friends, relatives, or colleagues who consistently show empathy and understanding. They're the people most likely to provide a supportive ear, a compassionate response, and even go the extra mile to further educate themselves about OCD (if you're having trouble identifying such people, take a peek at Chapter 7, which covers how to build and nurture social connections.) It might feel less overwhelming to start by sharing just a small part of your experience, allowing you to gauge others' reactions and see if you feel comfortable unveiling more personal information. You could also begin by confiding in a therapist or local OCD support group, which provides nonjudgmental opportunities to talk about your diagnosis.

Should I tell someone I'm dating? Deciding whether to disclose your disorder within the context of a romantic relationship requires an added layer of consideration because it can hinge on factors such as the level of established trust, the stage and seriousness of the relationship, and your own comfort with vulnerability. Trust is the bedrock here; you've got to feel confident in your partner's capacity for empathy and support before sharing such private aspects of your life. The *timing* also plays a pivotal role—while early dates may not be the right moment for such intimate disclosures, a relationship that is growing in depth and commitment may call for a higher degree of openness to foster true closeness and mutual understanding.

On one hand, revealing your OCD can pave the way for deeper connection and support, enhancing the strength of the bond with your partner. It offers them insight into your experiences and enables them to provide the understanding or assistance you might need. On the other hand, withholding this information can lead to misunderstandings and emotional strain, as maintaining a part of your life in secrecy can be challenging. Later in this chapter you'll find advice about choosing a private setting, providing a clear explanation of OCD, and being ready for questions. Chapter 9 explores strategies for flourishing in relationships while managing OCD. Consulting with a professional can offer further guidance tailored to your own situation, ensuring that whatever decision you make is in your best interest.

Should I tell people at work? Choosing whether to inform your boss or work colleagues about your OCD is another nuanced process. The culture of your workplace is one key element to consider. Environments that actively promote mental health awareness and provide support systems may be more receptive. It's also important to be aware of the legal protections in place, such as the Americans with Disabilities Act (ADA), that safeguard against discrimination. We'll return to this issue and other issues with OCD in the workplace in Chapter 10.

Your ability to be productive is yet another element to consider. If OCD symptoms are impacting your job performance, and you believe accommodations could help, sharing your diagnosis with your employer seems worthwhile. However, disclosure opens up the possibility of your OCD becoming public knowledge within the workplace, which could affect your work relationships and privacy. So carefully weigh the potential risks against the relief and support that may come from being open about your struggles. Disclosing your mental health status is not mandatory unless OCD directly affects your work and requires reasonable adjustments on the part of your employer. You might start by consulting with human resources (and a therapist) to understand the best approach and then prepare to talk to your boss, focusing on how the condition affects your work and what accommodations you might need.

WHEN AND WHERE?

By thoughtfully considering the timing and context of confiding in others, you'll create a supportive atmosphere that facilitates understanding and compassion, raising the likelihood of a rewarding experience. In particular, selecting the right moment to share your struggles with OCD can influence how your message is received and understood. I suggest choosing a time when both you and the person you are speaking with are calm and not preoccupied, ensuring that they are able to give you their full attention and are more likely to respond supportively. Definitely avoid times of high stress or conflict. Finally, make sure neither of you is in a rush. It can be difficult to know how long these conversations will last, and you don't want to be interrupted midstream.

Recognizing appropriate contexts and settings for disclosure is also important. I suggest you choose a private and comfortable setting, free from distractions and interruptions, that provides a safe environment for both you and the other person, fostering open communication and minimizing potential misunderstandings. Ensure that the setting is conducive to a meaningful conversation, where both parties can feel at ease expressing themselves and listening attentively.

SHOULD I USE SOCIAL MEDIA?

As you can probably sense, I recommend having this conversation in person, rather than via text or on social media. A face-to-face setting fosters personal connection, allowing for immediate empathy and support through nonverbal communication. It also affords more privacy, as you can control who receives the information directly from you. Furthermore, it increases clarity, reducing the chance of misunderstandings that can occur in text exchanges. Immediate feedback is another benefit, as it enables a real-time exchange of thoughts and emotions.

I understand, however, that electronic messages allow you to compose your thoughts at your own pace and reach a wider audience quickly. They also let you control the dialogue without immediate in-person reactions and provide an emotional cushion through the screen. Still, there are risks such as potential privacy breaches, the uncontrollable spread of information, a lack of instant support, the possibility that others will misinterpret what you're telling them, and the possibility that you will misinterpret others' responses to your communications because of the absence of verbal and nonverbal cues.

How to Craft Your Message

Clear communication is crucial when it comes to talking about OCD. The following strategies can help you get your message across clearly.

BE CLEAR AND CONCISE

Start by organizing your thoughts and pinpointing the key messages you want to convey. Aim for simplicity and clarity, avoiding overly complex explanations that could potentially lead to confusion. Write down what you want to say so that you stay on message, and practice beforehand—perhaps in front of a mirror or with a trusted friend—to refine your message and make sure it's easy to understand. Remember, the goal is to communicate your experience in a way that others can empathize with, creating a foundation for support and understanding.

USE "I" STATEMENTS

"I" statements are a powerful tool for expressing your personal experience with OCD. Saying "I feel . . . " or "I experience . . . " centers the conversation on your personal journey and helps you convey your thoughts and feelings in an authentic and relatable way. It also minimizes the potential for defensiveness from others because it focuses on your feelings rather than on placing blame or making assumptions about others' intentions or knowledge about OCD.

BE PREPARED FOR FAQS

FAQs are *frequently asked questions,* which are common queries that your audience may pose. It's wise to have some clear responses ready in advance. Here are some typical questions you might encounter, with suggested answers in italics:

- What is OCD (what are obsessions and compulsions)? *OCD stands for obsessive–compulsive disorder, a mental health condition characterized by persistent unwanted thoughts (obsessions), anxiety, and repetitive behaviors (compulsions).*

- How does it affect you? *(This question shows empathy and a willingness to understand your experience. Your response will vary depending on the nature of your OCD.)*

- What causes OCD, and how is it diagnosed? *The exact causes of OCD are unknown, but a combination of biological, psychological, and environmental factors is involved.*

- How can I support you? *Thank you! Showing that you understand me, avoiding judgment, and learning about OCD are the best things you can do to help me.*

- What triggers your symptoms? *(This question also shows compassion and a willingness to understand your OCD. Your response will vary depending on your symptoms.)*

- Is OCD treatable? What treatments work? Are you getting help, and if so, what kind? *There are certain psychological and medication treatments that can work. I am doing _____ therapy right now (or I am working on finding the best kind of help for me).*

- Does having OCD mean you're a perfectionist or like things extremely tidy? *While some people with OCD have symptoms related to perfectionism or cleanliness, these symptoms don't apply to everyone— OCD can appear in many different ways. For me, my obsessions concern _____ and my compulsive rituals are _____.*

Preparing answers to these kinds of questions in advance helps the conversation flow more smoothly and ensures that you're ready to provide informative and thoughtful responses. It is also empowering because it equips you with the tools to educate others about OCD and dispel potential misconceptions and stereotypes.

SET BOUNDARIES

Choosing to disclose your OCD is a personal decision, and it's important to establish in advance how much private information you're willing to share. When you're crafting your message, and before entering any conversation, think carefully about the level of detail you're comfortable with. Are you okay discussing your specific symptoms, the impact on your daily life, and the treatments you're pursuing? Or would you prefer to keep the dialogue focused on general information about OCD? Setting these boundaries beforehand will help you stay within your comfort zone and maintain control over how much of your private life becomes public knowledge. Keep in mind that once you've revealed your OCD to others, how far this information will travel is out of your hands. That's why I suggest having a mental script ready in order to stay focused and share only what feels right for you.

AVOID MEDICAL JARGON

While it's important to provide accurate information, keep your explanation easy to follow. Avoid using overly technical terms as they can create a barrier to understanding. Using plain language and relatable examples enhances the effectiveness of your message and ensures that your experience with OCD is conveyed clearly, authentically, and in a way that fosters empathy and support from others.

SOME SAMPLE SCRIPTS

Here are some sample scripts that reflect what I've discussed in this section. Feel free to use them as a guide if and when you decide to unveil your OCD to family and/or friends or in a professional setting. Notice the differences in these examples. The first script is casual, yet it sets a firm boundary about how much detail you're comfortable getting into. You might use script 2 if you're discussing your OCD with someone at work or school. Script 3, which is a bit warmer and more personal, might be appropriate with a friend or someone you're dating. Finally, notice that I suggest using the full name, *obsessive–compulsive disorder,* at first, to help avoid some of the trivializing and stigma around the term *OCD* (as in "you're so OCD").

    1. *Hey, I wanted to share something with you because I value our relationship. I have obsessive–compulsive disorder, which is something I deal with on a daily basis. While I'm open to talking about it in general, I'm not always comfortable going into all the details. I hope you understand that there are aspects of*

it that I prefer to keep private. But I do want you to know about it because it's a part of who I am.

2. *I think it's important for you to know that I have obsessive–compulsive disorder. It's something that I manage, and it doesn't define me, but it can affect how I function day to day. If it ever comes up in the context of my work or our interactions, I'm happy to explain how it might impact our project or my work flow. However, I prefer not to discuss the specifics of my experiences with it. Thank you for respecting my privacy in this matter.*

3. *I feel it's time I share something personal with you: I have obsessive–compulsive disorder. It's been a journey, and I've learned a lot about myself along the way. While I'm open to discussing what OCD is broadly, I hope you understand that I might not want to delve too deeply into my personal experiences with it. It means a lot to have your support and understanding, though.*

Responding to Reactions

When you decide to discuss your OCD with others, you'll want to prepare for a variety of responses—from deeply supportive to hopelessly uninformed. Some people may offer immediate understanding and empathy, recognizing OCD as the real problem that it is. Others, due to lack of awareness, might respond with confusion, emotionality, dismissiveness, or even inappropriate jokes. It's helpful to anticipate this spectrum of reactions and mentally rehearse how you might handle each of them. Always remember, the responses you receive reflect the other person's viewpoints and not your own experience.

APPRECIATING EMPATHY

Hopefully (and most likely), your disclosure will be met with genuine support and understanding. When it is, it's important to express gratitude. A response like "Thank you for being so understanding and supportive" acknowledges the other person's positive reaction. Sharing how their support impacts you, such as saying "Your reaction means a great deal to me and provides comfort," can deepen the connection. If they seem open, you might offer more information, either about your personal experiences or general facts, to enhance their understanding. If there are specific ways the other person can support you, this is a good opportunity to talk about them, like mentioning that you might need extra patience at times. Encourage ongoing dialogue and openness for future conversations and show your willingness to support the other person in return. This not only acknowledges the support you're receiving but also fosters a mutually respectful and understanding relationship.

HANDLING AN EMOTIONAL RESPONSE

If the other person becomes emotional, approach the situation with empathy and patience. Understand that this reaction may stem from concern, surprise, or a lack of understanding about OCD. So reassure the person and provide clarity. You might say something like "I see that this news has affected you, and I want you to know that it's okay. I'm still the same person I was before I told you about my OCD. This is just one part of who I am and doesn't define my entire being." Encourage an open dialogue in which the other person can express their feelings and ask questions. This can be an opportunity for both of you to learn from each other and strengthen your relationship.

ADDRESSING MISCONCEPTIONS

Dealing with misconceptions (for example, "Really? You have OCD? But you don't wash your hands a lot; you're actually pretty *messy*") and stigmatizing comments (such as "Mental disorders aren't real—they're just all in your head") are probably the most challenging aspect of disclosing your OCD. Stigma often arises from myths and misunderstandings about mental health conditions. One strategy is to have concise, factual information (like your responses to the previous FAQs) ready to share. Educating those around you can transform misconceptions into understanding. Keep resources at hand—whether it's literature or websites—that you can offer to those interested in learning more.

ENFORCING BOUNDARIES

As noted earlier in this chapter, if you find the conversation veering into territory you find too personal, or if someone asks questions that make you uncomfortable, you can redirect the dialogue. For example, you could steer the conversation back to a general discussion about OCD by saying something like "I think what's more important than my personal experience is the overall impact OCD has on people." Other conversational pivot points you might be prepared to use include "I appreciate your interest, but I'd prefer to talk about something else now" and "I'm not comfortable discussing these details; let's focus on _____." Remember that you're not obligated to share more than you want to, and it's okay to assert your limits at any time. Your story is yours to tell, and you have the right to choose how and when to tell it.

DEALING WITH DISRESPECT OR DISAPPROVAL

What if you encounter outright negative reactions? While this response can be disheartening, it also presents powerful opportunities to inform and enlighten someone about the realities of living with OCD. If you feel comfortable doing so, use these instances as teachable moments. Explain how comments or behaviors may be harmful or how certain stereotypes don't reflect your experience. But prioritize your own mental health! If a conversation becomes too confrontational or if you feel it's not the right moment, your best option is to end the conversation and seek support from someone who understands and can give you advice on how to proceed. Here are some courteous but clear closing statements you can use to enforce boundaries and signal the end of the discussion:

- Thank you for taking the time to listen, but I'd like to leave it here for now.
- I think we've covered a lot about my OCD. Let's switch topics and catch up on [another subject].
- It's been helpful to share some of my experiences, but I'm not comfortable continuing this part of the conversation. I'm sure you understand.

- If you're interested in learning more, I can recommend some great resources on OCD. For now, I'd prefer to talk about something a bit lighter.

- This conversation is getting a bit overwhelming for me, so I need to pause it here. Maybe we can talk more about it another time.

Seeking Help and Support

The complexities around letting others know about your OCD highlight the importance of a strong support system. Fortunately, there are numerous resources and support groups specifically tailored for people with OCD that can provide a community of understanding and shared experiences. Organizations such as the International OCD Foundation or IOCDF (*www.iocdf.org*) have directories of local support groups and online forums where you can seek connection and camaraderie with others who have experience opening up about OCD. Connecting with others who have walked a similar path can be an invaluable source of comfort and encouragement. In addition, there are individuals with OCD (or those who have successfully overcome the disorder) who maintain an active presence in the OCD community and provide peer support through interactive websites and one-on-one consultations. Hearing others share their stories and coping strategies can provide not just solace, but also practical advice for speaking with others about what you're going through. Of course, I cannot overstate the value of expert professional help in providing guidance on how to approach self-disclosure in a way that is healthy and beneficial for you.

Sharing your experience with OCD can be a powerful tool. It can help you erase feelings of isolation and shame and replace them with a greater sense of empowerment, self-acceptance, community, and shared experience. The validation and support that come from others can reinforce positive self-perception and contribute to a healthier, more optimistic outlook on life, which is a critical part of thriving with OCD. Not only that, but your story of OCD also adds to the collective understanding of the disorder, fostering greater societal awareness and acceptance. Indeed, personal narratives can challenge misconceptions and stereotypes, shedding more light on the reality of OCD. They, in turn, can lead to more compassionate attitudes and policies and a decrease in the stigma that so many people face.

I hope this chapter helps you feel equipped with the understanding and tools needed to navigate the delicate process of disclosing your OCD journey, should you decide to take this route. As you move forward, carry these insights with you and approach conversations about OCD with confidence, knowing that doing so can enrich your personal well-being. From support groups to professional help, you are surrounded by resources designed to assist and empower you on this journey to resilience and self-acceptance. In the next chapter, we'll delve deeper into how to enrich your social ties and connections to help you thrive with OCD.

Practical Steps for Living Well:
Finding a Balance between Privacy and Disclosure

Decide whether and to whom you want to disclose:

- Determine why you want to disclose having OCD and consider the pros and cons.
- Select friends, family, or colleagues who are supportive, trustworthy, and understanding.

Craft your disclosure carefully:

- Decide how much detail you'll share and write down (and practice) what you want to say.
- Choose a calm, private, and comfortable setting with plenty of time for the conversation.

When others respond supportively:

- Show gratitude.
- Describe specific ways they can support you.

If others respond negatively:

- Share factual information about OCD.
- Redirect or end the conversation if it veers into uncomfortable territory.

7

getting the healthy support you deserve

Living with intrusive thoughts, anxious feelings, and compulsive behaviors that other people don't seem to understand can feel like a lonely journey. But connecting with others gives you a sense of security and belonging, reducing feelings of isolation and providing encouragement and new perspectives to help you confront life with OCD. Building a social support network also helps distract you from obsessions and compulsions to lessen their hold. What's more, research shows that by increasing feelings of well-being, social support boosts your immune system and increases resilience to stress, thus reducing the risk of stress-related physical illnesses, such as heart disease and strokes.

This chapter delves into the role of support systems. You'll learn strategies for building and nurturing these essential connections. Various avenues for gaining support, including peer and professional networks as well as advocacy organizations, are described. You'll also get strategies for tackling obstacles associated with social support that often occur for people with OCD.

Harnessing the Power of a Social Support Network

When you're facing life with OCD, healthy social connections can enhance your journey by leading to greater satisfaction with life in numerous ways. Here are some of the key benefits:

- Reduced isolation
- Emotional support, empathy, and understanding from others
- Access to advice, new perspectives, and coping skills for managing tricky situations
- Resilience to anxiety, depression, and trauma
- Better cardiovascular health and a stronger immune system

Are you content with your social support network? If you find it lacking, this section offers guidance on how to enhance it.

Identifying Supportive People in Your Life

The first step is identifying those you can count on to reliably offer empathy and support. Look for friends, family members, coworkers, and acquaintances who show patience and a willingness to understand your experiences. Keep in mind that in finding supportive people quantity is less important than *quality*. You want people who listen without judgment, respect your boundaries, and offer encouragement. Consider doing the following to seek them out:

- **Reflect on past interactions:** Who has a good track record of being kindhearted and understanding in difficult times? Who are the good listeners that respond without judgment? Pay attention to how people react when you (or others) face challenges. Those who are patient and offer constructive support are likely good candidates.

- **Seek shared experiences:** People who have faced similar challenges (such as other mental health disorders) are often particularly empathic and supportive.

- **Consider trustworthiness:** Trust is crucial. Follow your intuition—do you feel comfortable and safe sharing your thoughts and experiences with the other person?

- **Look for emotional intelligence:** People who are good at understanding and managing their own feelings, as well as dealing with others' emotions, are often the most empathic and supportive.

- **Prioritize respect for boundaries:** Identify people who respect your boundaries and personal space, a crucial aspect of any supportive relationship.

The goal is to cultivate a network of people who make you feel heard, respected, and understood. So approach this process thoughtfully and choose people who make positive contributions to your well-being and ability to manage OCD. Once you've identified them, reach out with openness and honesty using the strategies covered in Chapter 6.

Cultivating Your Network

Building your social support network, however, is just the beginning. You also need to actively maintain it to ensure it continues to work effectively for you. It's a little like tending a garden: Just as a garden requires regular watering, weeding, and nurturing to thrive, your support network needs consistent effort, care, and dedication if you are to fully reap its benefits. Here's what you need to do.

COMMUNICATE

Consistent and open communication is the cornerstone of any strong relationship because it fortifies the bonds between people. Make it a point to stay in touch and share experiences through regular meetups, phone calls, or digital communication.

RECIPROCATE

If you rely on others for support, you've got to show up for them too. Listening, offering encouragement, and supporting those in your network by celebrating their successes and being there for them during tough times shows your investment in the relationship and cultivates a balanced and mutually rewarding connection where you both feel valued.

SHOW APPRECIATION

Let your supporters know you're grateful for what they do for you. This also deepens your connections and makes others want to step up in your times of need. Three excellent ways to show your appreciation are:

- **Verbal acknowledgments:** Telling someone directly how much you appreciate their support and understanding makes them feel valued. Let them know how they've positively impacted your life. Share your progress or moments of triumph so they can see the value of their support.

- **Acts of kindness:** Writing a thank-you note is a personal and heartfelt way to express gratitude. You could also give a gift to show your appreciation. Examples of appropriate gifts include a book, food basket, gift card, homemade item, or something you know has special significance for the person you want to thank.

- **Spending quality time together:** You can also show gratitude by enjoying activities together (such as cooking a meal, attending a festival, or playing a game) or just having a meaningful conversation. When you engage in shared interests, you not only strengthen your bond, but also receive a temporary distraction from the stress of OCD.

BE PATIENT AND FLEXIBLE

Life's constant changes affect people's availability and capacity to offer support. By being patient, you allow for understanding when others cannot provide immediate help. When you're flexible, you're able to modify how you engage with your network as circumstances evolve. This might mean changing communication methods (for example, phone calls instead of visits), adjusting the frequency of interactions, or redefining the roles different people play in your support system. For instance, if a friend who used to be your confidant becomes less available due to new responsibilities, you might need to seek additional support from other members of your network.

Leveraging Specialized Support from Peers and Groups

Although your social support network is great for offering general encouragement and companionship in various situations, you'll also gain from engaging in networks that provide specialized advice specifically designed for managing OCD. Peer support, provided by others living with OCD, can give you a unique understanding and shared perspective that your friends and family may lack. Advocacy groups, which are organizations dedicated to helping people affected by OCD, are also excellent sources of focused support. Fortunately, the OCD community is rich with support groups, peer support workers, and advocacy organizations the world over.

OCD Support Groups

In-person and online support groups offer environments for sharing experiences, feeling understood, and learning from others with OCD. There are online resources, including websites like the IOCDF (*www. iocdf.org*), that offer directories of both local and online support groups. Mental health clinics often provide information about regional groups and may even host their own. Social media platforms, such as Facebook and Reddit, also feature dedicated groups where people share experiences and advice. It's important when joining a group to make sure it aligns with your needs, so I recommend attending a few sessions to gauge the group's dynamics.

In-person support groups typically meet at a set location like a community center, treatment clinic, or even someone's home. Meetings are often scheduled on a weekly or monthly basis and are facilitated by an experienced group member. These groups provide a tangible sense of community and connection, allowing you to experience face-to-face interactions and support through activities such as discussions on specific topics, sharing personal experiences, and hearing from guest speakers. The physical presence of others who understand the challenges of OCD can be incredibly validating and comforting.

On the other hand, online support groups afford greater flexibility and accessibility, which might be important if you live in a rural area, have trouble getting around due to OCD symptoms, or simply prefer the anonymity of an online setting. These groups may operate through text posts, chat rooms, video meetings, or a combination of them. And since members might be online and active at various times throughout the day and night, they can offer a more consistent support system with quicker responses and interactions.

Peer Support Workers

Individual peer support workers, who have personal experience with OCD and are trained to support others with this disorder, can also play a role in helping you flourish. These people share their own journey, offering relatable insights and hope. By providing emotional support, they can help you feel less isolated and give suggestions for how to contend with the daily hassles caused by OCD. Peer support workers are also skilled at guiding you to useful resources, treatments, and support groups. As such, they can play a significant role in advocacy and empowerment, helping you take charge of your mental health. Websites like the IOCDF maintain lists of peer support workers, yet you can also find them by searching the internet more broadly and through referrals from professional therapists.

Advocacy Groups

Advocacy organizations can also play a pivotal role in your support. These associations have programs focusing on education, awareness, support, research, and public policy related to OCD and mental health more broadly. While the IOCDF, based in the United States, remains the flagship organization for OCD advocacy with affiliate groups in numerous states, there are similar organizations with the same mission in over 20 countries worldwide, including Canada, China, England, France, Nigeria, Norway, South Africa, Spain, and Sweden. Advocacy organizations also help bring together the OCD community by organizing events such as the IOCDF's annual OCD Conference and its One Million Steps for OCD Walk. These types of events offer opportunities to connect with others living with OCD, share experiences, and access the latest information about treatments and research. Becoming a member of an OCD advocacy organization is straightforward and comes with numerous benefits. By joining this organization, you gain access to a wealth of resources, including regular newsletters and exclusive online information and support. This membership not only connects you with a broader community, but also keeps you informed and supported in your journey.

Overcoming Obstacles to Seeking Support

Whether due to isolation, stigma, a lack of resources, or the presence of negativity, many people with OCD face significant obstacles in seeking the help and connections they need. Overcoming these barriers requires resilience and sometimes a creative approach to finding support in unexpected places.

Breaking the Cycle of Isolation

It's a vicious cycle: Social isolation exacerbates stress and anxiety, leading to more OCD symptoms and more isolation. To break out of this loop, you've got to actively seek supportive communities. Taking the initiative is key to forming meaningful connections, and involves actively reaching out and expressing interest in others, whether through starting conversations, inviting someone for coffee, or joining groups for people with common interests or concerns (such as support groups). This proactive approach sets the tone for mutual engagement and potentially leads to new friendships and stronger bonds. Although reaching out can be intimidating and carries the risk of rejection, the benefits of developing communication skills and building relationships often make it worthwhile, as many successful relationships start with one person taking that crucial first step.

SUPPORTIVE COMMUNITIES

Online forums and support groups are particularly beneficial as they provide a platform where you can interact with others who truly understand the challenges of living with OCD. As mentioned earlier, they also offer anonymity and accessibility, making it easier if you're hesitant to engage in face-to-face interactions or if OCD symptoms prevent you from doing so. Additionally, many of these groups organize regular virtual meetups, webinars, and discussion sessions, which can be a great source of continuous support.

PERSONAL RELATIONSHIPS

Maintaining and nurturing connections with friends and family are equally important. These relationships offer a different kind of support, grounded in personal history and emotional connection. Friends and family who are empathic and understanding can provide a sense of normality and stability, which is crucial for dealing with OCD. It's important to communicate openly with others about your needs and challenges, so you can help them understand how best to support you.

SOCIAL ACTIVITIES

Engaging in social activities also plays a significant role in preventing isolation. While doing so may feel daunting, especially during periods of heightened anxiety, participating in social events can provide a much-needed distraction and a sense of belonging. Activities can range from informal gatherings, like coffee meetups or walks in the park, to more structured events like book clubs or hobby groups. What's important is to find activities that are enjoyable and not too overwhelming.

ROUTINE SOCIAL INTERACTIONS

Finally, establishing a routine of regularly scheduled social interactions can provide a sense of structure and predictability. They might include weekly phone calls with a friend, family dinners, or regular attendance at a local support group. The regularity of these interactions can help create a rhythm in your life, making socializing less daunting and more a part of normal routine.

Tackling the Fear of Revealing OCD

Chapter 6 discussed the advantages and disadvantages of sharing your OCD diagnosis, as well as strategies for how to do so. However, actually taking the step to talk about OCD can feel scary, and your apprehension can intensify the stress and anxiety linked with obsessions and compulsions. Here are some strategies to help you effectively surmount these worries.

START WITH SOMEONE YOU TRUST

One of the most effective ways to begin addressing this fear is to confide in someone you know will look out for your interests and well-being, like a close friend or relative. This person should be someone who has shown understanding and empathy in the past. The act of sharing your experience with OCD can be liberating and can significantly reduce the burden of carrying this secret alone. Start by expressing your feelings and experiences and let them know why you are sharing this experience with them. Their support and understanding can be a strong foundation as you gradually acquire the confidence to open up to a wider circle.

EXPAND YOUR CIRCLE GRADUALLY

As you become more comfortable discussing OCD-related issues, consider slowly expanding the circle of people you share this information with. Sharing more widely doesn't mean you have to tell everyone; rather, it's about identifying people you believe will be supportive—friends, colleagues, classmates, or fellow members of your support group. Each positive experience of sharing your story boosts your confidence and lessens your fear.

BE PREPARED FOR RESPONSES AND REACTIONS

As discussed in Chapter 6 (in the section "Responding to Reactions"), prepare for questions or reactions people might have when you tell them about OCD. Think about common misconceptions and how you might address them. Preparing a few key points or facts to talk about can help you feel more in control. And remember, you are not obligated to answer every question. It's okay to set boundaries regarding what you are comfortable discussing.

PRACTICE SELF-COMPASSION AND ASSERTIVENESS

Remind yourself that having OCD is not something to be ashamed of—it's a *part* of who you are, but it does not *define* you. Practicing self-compassion (as I described in Chapter 2) helps reduce feelings of fear and shame associated with disclosure. It's also important to be assertive about your rights. You have the autonomy to decide when, how, and to whom you disclose your OCD. If you encounter negative reactions, remind yourself that your openness is a sign of your strength and that not everyone may understand immediately. There's more about responding to negative reactions a bit later in this chapter.

SEEK PROFESSIONAL SUPPORT

If the fear of revealing your OCD feels overwhelming, consider seeking support from a mental health professional. Therapists can provide you with tailored strategies to manage this fear and can also help you practice discussing OCD.

Breaking Free from Embarrassment and Stigma

Do feelings of embarrassment or the fear of social stigma hold you back from seeking and embracing the healthy social support you need?

Here's what you can do to overcome these challenges and build a supportive network.

EDUCATE YOURSELF AND OTHERS

Knowledge is the most powerful antidote to stigma. As already explained, educating yourself about OCD bolsters your confidence in discussing it with others. Understanding the nature of obsessions and compulsions, their prevalence, and the fact that OCD is a recognized mental health condition can help mitigate feelings of shame. Sharing this knowledge with those in your social circle can also foster a more understanding and supportive environment. When others understand what OCD entails, they're more likely to offer empathy rather than judgment.

PRACTICE SELF-COMPASSION

Flip back to Chapter 2 and make sure you're applying the strategies for developing self-compassion. Treating yourself with kindness and understanding and recognizing that OCD is not a flaw or weakness are absolutely essential to eliminating embarrassment as a barrier to developing your support network. Remember that OCD is a challenge many people face. Seeking help is a sign of strength, not weakness.

SEEK GUIDANCE

Here again, help from a mental health professional or OCD support worker can be instrumental. Clinicians and others trained to understand OCD can give you specific techniques to change negative thought patterns and enhance your self-esteem. They can also provide guidance on how to effectively communicate your needs and experiences to others, making the process of seeking support less daunting.

CREATE SAFE SPACES FOR CONNECTION

Actively seeking out supportive communities, whether online or in person, can significantly help in overcoming the barriers of embarrassment and stigma. Support groups for people with OCD can provide a sense of belonging and understanding. In these spaces, sharing

experiences with others who have faced similar challenges can normal-
ize your experiences and reduce feelings of isolation.

Navigating through Negativity

Unfortunately, at some point in your journey with OCD it's likely
you'll encounter unhelpfulness and disapproval. When dealing with
people who are critical, judgmental, or otherwise unsupportive, you'll
want to assess how much influence they have in your life so you can
minimize their impact. If someone is especially detrimental to your
well-being, it may be necessary to limit or end contact with them by
setting clear boundaries. In cases where avoiding interactions isn't possible, you'll want to find ways to focus on your own self-care despite
the negativity. Here are some methods for putting your well-being first
and steering clear of negative energy.

IDENTIFY YOUR "DOWNERS"

"Downers" are the people in your life who tend to lower your morale
through their negative comments, pessimism, disapproval, criticism,
or generally discouraging behavior. I'd be willing to bet you already
know who your downers are. If not, identifying them is important
because your interactions with them can significantly impact your
journey toward living well with OCD. These unsupportive individuals might be acquaintances, family members, or colleagues who fail to
understand the complexities of OCD, contributing to feelings of isolation and discouragement. Think through these two questions:

1. Who are the people whose mere presence, or even the thought
   of being around them, has the power to put you in a sour mood?
2. How much do these people, and their negativity, impact your
   life?

REDEFINE THE PROBLEM

In situations where you encounter subtle or unintentional negativity
that has little impact on you, the most helpful thing is often just a shift

in perspective: Remind yourself that the issue lies with the downer, not with you! Maybe they're dealing with personal issues of their own or haven't learned to think carefully about how their behavior affects others. In such instances, it might not be worth your time and energy to respond to the behavior at all. Instead, simply changing your viewpoint creates a mental buffer for yourself, which significantly reduces the stress and emotional impact of the negativity. You're acknowledging that while you can't control the downer's behavior, you *can* control how you make sense of it. This strategy can be a powerful tool in maintaining your well-being, especially in situations where you can't avoid interactions with downers. It helps you navigate through the situation with minimal stress and stay focused on your own wellness.

SET LIMITS AND BOUNDARIES

On the other hand, in cases where the impact is more significant, responding by setting clear boundaries becomes necessary. This might involve limiting your interactions with the person or, in some cases, ending the relationship. Setting boundaries is not a sign of weakness but a form of self-care and an assertion of your needs. Clear communication about these boundaries is key. Express the impact that the person's behavior has on you, being as direct yet as respectful as possible. Here are several examples of what you might say:

- I want to talk about something important. When you [describe specific behavior or action], it triggers my OCD symptoms. I need us to find a different way to handle this situation, so it's less stressful for me.

- I've noticed that our discussions about [specific topic] often leave me feeling anxious and worsen my OCD symptoms. I need to avoid these topics to keep my stress levels manageable. Let's focus our conversations on different subjects.

- I need your understanding of my OCD rituals. Commenting on them or rushing me makes my life harder. Please allow me the time I need to do these things, even if they seem unusual to you.

- I know you mean well with your suggestions about managing

my OCD, but sometimes it can be overwhelming. I'm following professional advice, so let's focus *our* conversations on other
topics.

- When you make comments like [specific example], they can be
  hurtful and exacerbate my OCD symptoms. I'd appreciate it if
  we could avoid making light of my condition.

- I want to clear up some common misunderstandings about
  OCD. It's not just about being neat or orderly. When we talk
  about it, I'd appreciate it if we could stick to facts and avoid stereotypes, because I find them damaging.

- There are times when I need to be alone to manage my OCD
  symptoms. During these times I'd appreciate some space. I'll
  reach out when I'm ready to interact again.

Each of these examples shows how to communicate your needs
clearly and directly, yet respectfully, with the understanding that the
other person may not fully grasp the complexities of living with OCD.
The goal is to create a supportive environment where you can manage
your condition effectively without additional stress from interpersonal
interactions. It may also be helpful to seek support from a therapist or
counselor when preparing for and having these conversations.

USE TACT WITH AUTHORITY FIGURES

But what if your downer holds a position of power—such as a boss or
teacher—and it's impossible to avoid interactions with them? Dealing
with these situations requires a tactful approach that balances assertive-
ness with respect for authority. To this end, it's important to maintain
professionalism and use "I" statements to express how the negativity affects you, with a statement such as, "I feel overwhelmed when I
consistently receive negative feedback." You can also seek clarification
on their comments to understand their perspective better and focus
on problem solving rather than on direct confrontation; for example,
you could say something like "I appreciate your input. Could you
please provide some specific examples so I can better understand your
perspective?" If necessary, request a private meeting to discuss your

concerns and document any incidents in which their behavior adversely affects your work. Then, if applicable, seek advice from the human resources department or a trusted confidant or professional. If the situation doesn't improve, you might decide to consider your long-term goals and whether your work or school environment is the best one for your growth.

Navigating unsupportive relationships is a complex but essential aspect of achieving a satisfying quality of life with OCD. By assessing the influence of unsupportive individuals, setting boundaries, focusing on your own progress, engaging in self-care, and prioritizing your mental health, you can create a more supportive and understanding environment conducive to feeling fulfilled.

From identifying empathic individuals to nurturing these relationships and managing interactions with unsupportive people, this chapter has equipped you with strategies to build a resilient support system. Remember, establishing and maintaining healthy connections are key to reducing isolation, enhancing well-being, and lessening the grip of OCD symptoms. People you are already close to can be your biggest supporters, but as you probably know, within family settings you also have to deal with delicate dynamics. In Chapter 8 we explore how to disentangle the disorder's impact on family life and foster a supportive and understanding home environment.

Practical Steps for Living Well:
Getting the Healthy Support You Deserve

Identify your support network:

- Include people who have been kind, understanding, and patient with you.
- Schedule regular check-ins, but be patient, flexible, and appreciative.

Break the cycle of isolation:

- Actively seek out supportive communities and social activities.
- Engage in regular social interactions.

Tackle the fear of revealing OCD:

- Confide in someone you trust and gradually expand your circle of disclosure.
- Prepare for potential questions and responses about your experience with OCD.

Navigate through negativity:

- Set boundaries to prevent the "downers" in your life from lowering your morale.
- Focus on problem solving rather than on confrontation.

8

maintaining family harmony

As you already know, obsessional fears and compulsive rituals affect not only you but your whole household, influencing family routines, emotions, and the overall well-being of family members. To address these challenges, you need communication strategies that will foster an environment of empathy and mutual understanding. In this chapter we'll delve into techniques for articulating feelings and thoughts and for actively listening to your relatives' perspectives. This will pave the way for collaborative problem solving, focusing on tailored approaches that consider the unique needs and constraints of each family member. Through this comprehensive approach, you and your family can work together to navigate the complexities of living with OCD, striving for a balanced and supportive home life.

Understanding Your OCD in the Family Context

Becoming aware of how your OCD symptoms affect family dynamics is the first step toward working together to manage the disorder while also keeping family life balanced. A central feature of OCD is the intense need to feel safe, which, in a family setting, can unintentionally lead to family members becoming involved in rituals and other OCD-related behaviors. One way in which this happens is allowing the family's routines to be dictated by your efforts to alleviate obsessional fears. For instance, if you have obsessions about contamination, you might ask family members to adhere to certain cleaning protocols. Additionally, family members may instinctively assist with your rituals and avoidance behaviors, not because you've asked them to, but out of a desire to ease your distress. In these scenarios, your OCD transforms from a personal challenge into a shared family experience, with family members becoming part of your coping mechanism. Such dynamics can strain the family environment, causing frustration and tension as your loved ones grapple with the demands and limitations imposed by OCD.

Here are some additional ways OCD can impact family life. As you go through these descriptions, consider how each one might be present in your own household or within your extended family.

• **Interference with routines:** Compulsive rituals can disrupt daily family activities and schedules. For instance, a family dinner might be delayed due to lengthy cleaning rituals. Bedtime routines may be prolonged owing to repeated checking behaviors. Work might be interrupted to answer repeated requests for reassurance. These disruptions can lead to frustration and inconvenience as family members adjust their routines and other plans to accommodate rituals.

• **Emotional stress:** Living alongside your OCD symptoms can be emotionally challenging for your family members. They might feel unsure of how to help or react to your obsessional thoughts and anxiety. Their involvement in your rituals, reassurance seeking, and avoidance can create a tense and sometimes confrontational atmosphere. This ongoing stress can lead to feelings of frustration and resentment, affecting the overall well-being of the family.

• **Misunderstandings and conflicts:** Your family members might find your OCD symptoms perplexing or illogical, potentially leading them to mistakenly view your behaviors as being stubborn, lazy, or inconsiderate. For example, a parent might feel disrespected if their child is constantly late for family activities because they're stuck performing compulsive rituals. Children might feel confused and upset if a parent's OCD symptoms seem frightening or overly restrictive. These misunderstandings can lead to conflicts, arguments, and strained relationships within the family.

• **Increased responsibility for others:** To accommodate the demands of OCD, other family members may end up with extra responsibilities around the house, such as taking over household chores that you can't perform because of obsessional fears or stepping in to manage aspects of daily life that are disrupted by rituals. Over time asking others to do your chores can lead to an imbalance in the distribution of tasks and responsibilities, placing an unfair burden on some family members and leading to feelings of resentment.

• **Social limitations:** OCD can also affect the family's social life. Does your family avoid social gatherings and other events to prevent exposure to fear triggers? Do they refrain from inviting guests over? This behavior can lead to isolation for you and other family members, limiting opportunities for social interaction, support, and entertainment and potentially contributing to feelings of frustration, loneliness, and disconnection from the broader community.

Family Impact Journaling

To deepen your understanding of how your OCD affects family dynamics and to prepare for resolving any conflicts, I suggest keeping a journal for one week in which you note instances when your OCD symptoms have impacted family life as I've described. For instance, write about a time when your checking rituals delayed a family outing or when your need for reassurance led to a tense conversation. Alongside each incident, record your own feelings and perceptions, as well as those of your family members. For example, you could note your frustration at not being understood or the apparent stress or confusion in a family member. After a week, review your journal entries to identify patterns. Are there particular situations or times of day when conflicts arise? Are certain family members more affected than others?

Productive Family Communication Patterns

Once you've identified the effects of OCD on your family, you can begin addressing these issues through open conversation and collaborative problem solving. However, navigating these discussions effectively requires specific communication techniques, including clearly articulating your own thoughts and feelings, actively listening to what your family members have to say, and working together to implement possible solutions. These skills both help resolve OCD-related complications and also foster stronger, more supportive relationships. In fact, as you'll see in later chapters, these communication strategies serve as a foundation for navigating the interplay between OCD and various other types of interpersonal dynamics. So let's explore them in detail.

Sharing Thoughts and Feelings

There are strategic ways to let your loved ones in on what you're thinking and feeling—whether it's an obsessional fear or feelings of frustration over a lack of support. When you express what's on your mind in a polite, open, and honest way, it enhances empathy and leads to mutual understanding and greater cooperation. Here are some guidelines for effectively sharing your thoughts and feelings with your family (you might encourage other family members to use them too).

OWN HOW YOU FEEL

Remember the "I" statements that were introduced in Chapter 6? Here's another place where they're important. When speaking with family members, try stating your thoughts and fears from your own perspective rather than as absolute truths. For example, instead of stating, "Thirteen is an unlucky number, and we all have to avoid it," try, "I feel anxious when the number 13 shows up because it triggers my OCD." Make sure to be open and clear about how you *feel* when a particular situation affects you. For instance, "I feel hurt when my fear of bad luck isn't taken seriously," or "I feel loved and supported when you help me through my OCD rituals." Try not to use the word *you,* especially if it will put the other person on the defensive (as in "I'm angry that *you* don't take me seriously"); instead include something positive, like "While I'm grateful for the patience you usually show me, right now I'm angry that I'm not being taken seriously."

BE SPECIFIC

When you're specific and clear about your thoughts and feelings, your family members can better understand exactly where you're coming from—and that's the whole idea. For example, "I get anxious when I can't follow my daily routine, especially because it makes my OCD symptoms worse" is specific and informative. In contrast, "I feel bad today" is not.

SPEAK IN PARAGRAPHS

Share your thoughts in manageable "chunks." After expressing a main idea, pause to give the other person a chance to absorb what you're saying and respond. This way of speaking prevents you from overwhelming them with too much information at once and encourages a dialogue, which strengthens your relationship.

TACT AND TIMING

Be mindful of how and when you express your thoughts and feelings. Choose a moment when your family member is likely to be receptive and frame your concerns in a way that's respectful and nonconfrontational. For instance, choosing a calm, relaxed time to discuss a difficult situation and using a gentle tone can make it easier for the other person to listen and respond to what you have to say without becoming defensive.

Active Listening

Active listening involves being fully present when your family members are speaking to you. This means paying complete attention and avoiding any distractions so you can focus on what they're saying without letting your mind wander to other thoughts, such as how you're going to respond. Here are some important dos and don'ts.

UNDERSTAND AND ACKNOWLEDGE

The main task of active listening is to put yourself in the other person's shoes and try to understand their perspective—*even if you don't share the same viewpoint.* Listening to and understanding someone else's point of view is not the same thing as agreeing with them. Separating your family member's perspective from your own beliefs or judgments is critical for a healthy exchange of thoughts and feelings, even amid differing opinions. Your job is simply to listen and learn where the other person is coming from.

USE NONVERBAL BEHAVIOR

Use your body to show that you're engaged in the conversation and listening to what the other person has to say. Here are some ways to send powerful unspoken messages that you're tuned in:

- Nodding to signify understanding
- Maintaining eye contact to show attentiveness
- Uncrossing your arms to communicate receptiveness
- Leaning in slightly to indicate interest in what the other person is saying
- Using a range of facial expressions in response to the other person's words (for example, a look of concern when they are sharing something distressing or a smile when they share something positive)

REFLECT AND CLARIFY

When your family member is finished expressing an idea, summarize their feelings, desires, conflicts, and thoughts back to them to ensure that you understood their point and to show that you're genuinely listening and following the conversation. For instance, if a family member says, "I don't like it when you ask a million questions at dinner about how I'm preparing the food we eat. No one else can get a word in edgewise, and it feels like you don't trust me," you could say something like "I get that you're frustrated that I ask you lots of questions during dinner. You feel like I don't trust you and that my compulsions ruin our family time. Do I have that right?"

RESPOND THOUGHTFULLY

Once you've shown that you understand the other person's point, respond in a way that acknowledges their thoughts and feelings. Be sure your response is respectful and constructive—*even if the other person hasn't been*. For example, "I see how upsetting my compulsive questioning is for you, and I don't want to ruin dinnertime for our family. Let's think together about ways to manage these times more effectively." This approach validates the other person's experience, shows understanding, and offers constructive support, all of which are crucial in nurturing a supportive family environment when you have OCD.

AVOID THESE BAD HABITS

When a family member is misunderstanding or criticizing you, there's a temptation to interrupt and set them straight. But don't! This response only leads to escalated conflicts and more hurt feelings, hindering the opportunity for mutual understanding and effective problem solving. Here are some particular types of responses to avoid:

- Asking questions (other than to clarify the other person's perspective) like "Do you even think about how many germs there are on the cutting board?"
- Expressing your own viewpoints prematurely; for instance, "But I can't help it. I have OCD!"
- Interpreting or altering the meaning of the other person's statements, such as "So, you're saying you don't want me around for dinner anymore."

- Judging or correcting what the speaker has said, such as "You're wrong. No one else minds that I ask questions at dinner."

- Trying to negotiate or solve the problem right then and there; for instance, "So how about if you just promise me that you'll wash your hands with soap each time you touch the cutting board?"

You probably noticed that simply sharing thoughts and feelings or practicing active listening doesn't inherently lead to resolving issues like how to allocate household tasks, make decisions about participation in social events, or manage schedules around compulsive rituals. But these strategies are very important because they lay the groundwork for working together to find and implement solutions. I can't emphasize this enough: You and your family will only succeed in having more solution-focused discussions, as outlined in the next section, after building a solid foundation of understanding with these skills.

Problem Solving and Decision Making

After ensuring that both you and your family members fully understand each other's perspective, a good way to transition into a more solution-focused discussion is to ask, "Are we ready to work toward a solution now?" Then follow the guidelines provided next for an effective approach to decision making.

CLARIFY THE ISSUE

Start by identifying the problem. For instance, "I'd like to talk about how we can work together so I can limit my reassurance seeking at dinnertime." Then each person should share their understanding of the issue and explain why it matters to them—but without suggesting solutions yet. For instance, you might say, "I get worried that you don't pay enough attention to all the ways that food can become contaminated during meal preparation and that we could all get sick. I realize it's my OCD, but I'm still afraid that it could happen. That's what leads to all of my reassurance-seeking questions when we sit down to eat dinner."

Use active listening skills to let the other person share their thoughts about the issue as well.

BRAINSTORM SOLUTIONS

Then move on to thinking about possible solutions. But be sure to focus on ideas for what can be done differently in the future, rather than trying to figure out who is right or wrong. Also at this stage the goal is for everyone to brainstorm a range of potential solutions, without immediately judging their feasibility or acceptability. Feel free to propose any ideas, no matter how unworkable they might seem. You'll refine and evaluate the suggestions in the next step, where a mutually agreeable way forward will be selected. Sticking with the example of obsessions about food poisoning, here are some possible solutions:

- Have a family meeting where we watch educational videos about safe food handling practices, expiration dates, and proper cooking temperatures; then create guidelines for preparing food at home.
- Involve me in food preparation to increase my comfort with and knowledge of the process.
- Create a list of foods I feel safe eating and try to serve them.
- Set a limit on the number of reassurance-seeking questions that will be answered.
- Use visual aids in the kitchen for food safety, like color-coded cutting boards.
- Schedule meals so I know in advance what to expect and can prepare my own food.

DECIDE ON A SOLUTION AND TEST IT OUT

Now once you've explored options, choose a solution that seems agreeable to all parties, is respectful of each family member's needs and perspectives, and is workable in your family. Compromises are usually necessary, which means the solution will probably not align perfectly with your (or others') initial expectations. For example, you and your family might agree on a certain limit for reassurance-seeking questions, which may be less than you ideally wanted (and more than other family members would prefer); but it's a middle ground that works for everyone involved. Make sure the decision is specific and realistic, avoiding choices that could lead to resentment or are unlikely to be followed through.

Last, conduct a test run of the new approach to evaluate its success. Be prepared to give it some time, adjusting as necessary, to make it work. For instance, agree to try the new reassurance-seeking limit for a week and then discuss its success and how it's impacting your own well-being and family dynamics. If everyone agrees the solution is working, keep using it. If not, go back to the drawing board and try working out another possible way forward.

Managing More Serious OCD-Related Family Conflicts

The strategies for sharing thoughts and feelings, active listening, problem solving, and decision making will help you and your family navigate many challenges that arise either directly or indirectly from OCD symptoms. However, when faced with more serious conflicts rooted in the complexities of this disorder, you might require a more tailored approach. In this section I'll lead you through a series of steps aimed at effectively handling these situations and promptly resolving conflicts as they arise. Although the foundational communication strategies already discussed will play a large role in resolving such conflicts, you'll need to integrate additional tactics and considerations.

Identify Triggers

Serious family conflict related to OCD can arise from different sources, often related to the nature of symptoms and their impact on family life. For example, does your insistence that family members follow certain rules, assist with your rituals, or abide by other OCD-driven routines cause significant friction in your household? The first step in managing conflicts related to OCD is to identify the specific triggers that lead to tension within your family. Other common sources of conflict include:

- **Misunderstandings:** Family members might not fully understand OCD, leading to misconceptions about why you behave in certain ways. For example, they might believe it's just laziness or that using simple logic will help you "snap out of it." This lack of understanding can result in frustration and impatience.

- **Accommodation:** Driven by the desire to minimize your distress, family members may alter their routines or take on extra responsibilities. Although this approach might help alleviate *your* distress (at least in the moment), your family members may resent the constant adjustments and the added burden it places on their daily lives, leading to a sense of imbalance and potential frustration within the family unit. For example, consistently giving in to reassurance-seeking behaviors might become burdensome and frustrating over time.

- **Disruption of daily routines:** OCD rituals and compulsions can disrupt family routines and schedules. If you consistently require excessive time to complete tasks, delaying family activities or plans, the result might lead to inconvenience and strain for everyone involved.

- **Communication breakdown:** Miscommunication or lack of effective communication about the emotional and tangible needs and challenges of living with OCD can lead to misunderstandings and conflicts.

- **Emotional stress:** OCD can be emotionally draining for family members, leading to feelings of frustration, exhaustion, or even resentment.

- **Financial pressure:** The costs associated with OCD symptoms, such as spending money on specific cleaning supplies, on replacement items for those that have been discarded, on higher utility bills, and even for continued medication or therapy, can create financial stress and disagreements within the family.

- **Social limitations:** Avoidance of social gatherings can limit the family's social life, leading to feelings of isolation or frustration.

• **Role changes and imbalances:** The family dynamics might shift to accommodate your needs, leading to imbalances in roles and responsibilities that can create tension.

Do you recognize any of these sources of conflict in your family? If so, start by writing them down in a journal and describing how they play a role. Doing so will help you prepare for "high-risk" situations when you'll need to employ effective communication strategies, anticipate potential triggers, and proactively manage your responses in a way that minimizes conflict and promotes understanding within your family. This preparation can be crucial in navigating these challenging moments with greater awareness and control.

Communicate Effectively

When conflict arises, begin by applying the communication skills introduced earlier in this chapter—namely, sharing thoughts and feelings and active listening. Let's say one of your family members becomes aggravated because your rituals are making the whole family late for events. Effective communication involves fully absorbing and understanding their concerns and then offering your perspective. Encourage them to share their thoughts and feelings as you attend carefully to what they're saying, showing that you genuinely grasp the source of their frustration (even if you disagree). You might say something like "I see how my rituals cause us to be late, and I understand this is really frustrating for you." Resist the temptation to justify your behavior or offer a quick fix—you will have the opportunity to express your feelings and needs shortly. For now, it's about showing the other person that you genuinely understand and acknowledge their feelings. This alone can often help de-escalate conflict because it reduces defensiveness and paves the way for problem solving.

De-Escalation Strategies

Once your family member's concerns have been expressed and understood, begin working toward problem solving and decision making. But use these strategies for de-escalating conflict, minimizing family tension, and fostering better understanding.

PAY ATTENTION TO YOUR TONE

Make sure to maintain a calm and even tone of voice during discussions—even if you're frustrated. This keeps the conversation productive and respectful.

STICK TO "I" STATEMENTS

Make sure to express your feelings and needs from your personal perspective, rather than placing blame or making accusatory statements. For example, in a situation in which a family member unknowingly disrupts your OCD ritual, saying "*I* feel anxious and unsettled when my ritual is interrupted unexpectedly" is more constructive than accusingly stating "*You* always interrupt me and don't respect my needs."

AVOID FINGER POINTING

Blaming family members makes them feel defensive and leads to a more heated argument. Instead focus on expressing how the situation affects you and what could be done differently. For example, if a family member's action provokes an obsession, instead of blaming them for your heightened anxiety, try calmly explaining the trigger and discussing how to avoid such situations in the future.

SEEK A COMPROMISE

Use the problem-solving and decision-making strategies discussed earlier in this chapter to find a middle ground that addresses both your and your family's needs. For instance, if your cleaning rituals are time-consuming, compromising might involve scheduling these rituals at times that are less disruptive to family activities.

USE A MEDIATOR

In some situations, the conflict may become so challenging that it's difficult to resolve within your family. In such instances, involving someone from outside the immediate family—another relative, a friend, or

a therapist—can be beneficial. A mental health professional, in particular, is trained to mediate such conversations and can offer an objective
viewpoint and guide the family toward identifying underlying issues,
facilitating understanding, and working toward solutions that are con-
siderate of everyone's needs.

It's important to understand that using these communication and
de-escalation strategies is not about accepting all of the blame, dis-
regarding your own needs, or letting others silence you. Instead, it's
a strategic approach to managing conflict effectively. By actively listening and demonstrating empathy, you help to reduce defensiveness
and create a more collaborative environment. This approach allows
for a more productive dialogue, in which everyone's concerns can be
addressed. There's no shame in taking the high road to de-escalate ten-
sions; in fact, it shows strength and maturity. Doing so paves the way
for meaningful problem solving and the development of lasting solutions that respect and consider the needs of all involved.

We have explored the many ways OCD affects family life and
the importance of effective communication strategies to manage these
challenges. The tools and techniques covered in this chapter are essential stepping-stones toward a more harmonious environment and will
often be sufficient to restore family functioning despite the presence
of your OCD symptoms. Keep in mind, however, that it's impossible
to fully avoid family stress and conflict. Some level of disagreement
is normal in any family—and especially those affected by OCD. So
instead of trying to avoid confrontation altogether, focus on managing
disagreements respectfully in a supportive way. By identifying triggers,
practicing healthy communication strategies, and using conflict resolution techniques, you and your family can navigate the complexities
of living with OCD more effectively. If you have a romantic partner,
you know that OCD influences intimate relationships as well. The
next chapter explores how to prevent obsessions and compulsions from
overshadowing your romantic life.

Practical Steps for Living Well:
Maintaining Family Harmony

Educate your family:

- Help your relatives understand your experience and challenges.
- Hold family meetings to find collaborative solutions for OCD-related issues.

Practice good communication skills:

- Use "I" statements to express your feelings and needs without blaming others.
- Encourage family members to use active listening techniques.
- Be willing to compromise when finding solutions to problems.

Target accommodation:

- Identify accommodation behaviors in your family.
- Develop a plan with family members to gradually reduce accommodation.

Share pleasant activities:

- Participate in fun activities together to strengthen your family bond.
- Schedule regular family activities to extend interactions beyond OCD.

9

thriving in romantic relationships

Embarking on the adventure of a relationship while navigating the turbulent waters of OCD can feel like steering a ship through a storm. Your heart desires closeness, yet OCD looms like an uninvited third wheel, casting shadows on your romantic aspirations. The distressing and time-consuming nature of obsessions, avoidance, and compulsive rituals can hinder dating, emotional connections, trust, and physical intimacy, reducing your ability to enjoy shared experiences or maintain a sense of normality with a partner. This chapter delves into the heart of these challenges, offering practical strategies to help you foster close personal connections that are resilient against the tide of OCD whether you're taking tentative steps in a new relationship or nurturing a long-standing bond.

Chapter 6 laid out the considerations around disclosing your OCD to someone you're dating or in a relationship with. The material in this chapter is applicable whether or not you've shared this aspect of your life, although some approaches will be more effective if your partner is aware and understanding of your OCD. If you haven't discussed this topic, you might revisit Chapter 6, which provides guidance (in the section "Who Should I Tell?") on how to open up about OCD.

How Does OCD Affect Relationships?

The techniques and practices offered in this chapter are designed to help you overcome any obstacles to good intimate relationships that OCD may impose, paving the way for a more fulfilling romantic journey. The first step is to understand the different ways that OCD can impact intimate relationships. This knowledge allows you to then think about whether, and how, each potential impact relates to you. The numerous possibilities that are described next may leave you feeling some dismay about your love life, but keep in mind that knowledge is power and equips you to find ways to live well in your romantic relationship despite OCD's tendency to interfere. Knowing what you're experiencing is key here, so don't just *think* about this; keep a journal to record your thoughts and experiences.

OBSESSIONAL FEARS

Different types of obsessions present unique obstacles to dating and romantic relationships. Fears of contamination (such as from sexually transmitted infections) can obviously lead you to feel anxious and to avoid physical contact, creating barriers to emotional and physical intimacy as well as misunderstandings between you and your partner. If you have harm-related obsessions, you might feel an urge to be excessively cautious or to anxiously ask if your partner feels safe, leading to confusion and frustration for both of you. Intrusive and distressing obsessions about sex, including taboo thoughts and images, may not only ruin the mood during intimate moments but also spark worries about whether you've betrayed your partner. Finally, *relationship OCD* (ROCD) involves obsessional doubts concerning the "rightness" of your relationship, leading to a continuous need for reassurance and resulting in misunderstandings and diminishing trust. This rundown may feel like a lot to take in —but solutions follow.

COMPULSIVE BEHAVIORS

It's not difficult to imagine how disruptive excessive or untimely washing and cleaning might be to spontaneity in romantic and sexual encounters. A partner who knows that you experience such compulsions may also feel pressured to adapt to stringent cleanliness standards and end up resenting this pressure. Checking compulsions like repeatedly seeking reassurance from your partner can erode trust and also create frustration over the time and focus they require. Mental rituals, like analyzing and praying, can distance partners emotionally and hinder the depth and quality of your interactions. Last, compulsively confessing unwanted thoughts that might upset your partner—such as unwelcome ideas of cheating on your partner or acting violently toward them—can lead to distress and confusion, adversely affecting the trust and overall well-being of your relationship.

ACCOMMODATION

Has your partner taken over chores you avoid for OCD-related reasons? Do they limit *their* activities or social interactions to prevent triggering *your* obsessional fears? These kinds of adjustments might be well intended, and they might temporarily help keep your anxiety under control, but they can also strain your relationship. Specifically, when your partner helps with avoidance or your compulsions, it can end up interfering with routine tasks, upsetting the balance of shared responsibilities, and reducing your partner's trust in you and their sense of autonomy and independence.

SEXUAL DYSFUNCTION

When you're anxious, the body releases hormones like cortisol and adrenaline that put you in a state of fight or flight. Among the many changes that occur during this response is a reduction of blood flow to the genitals. In men this can contribute to difficulties achieving or maintaining an erection, and in women it can lead to decreased lubrication and reduced sexual responsiveness. Furthermore the worry over these effects can heighten performance anxiety, worsening the problem and fueling a self-perpetuating cycle: anxiety causes sexual difficulties, which then amplifies the anxiety about performance. Over time this cycle can lead a couple to shy away from physical intimacy.

STRAIN ON COMMUNICATION

Your partner might misinterpret your constant fear or need for reassurance as a sign of distrust. Avoidance of physical intimacy can result in feeling rejected. Obsessive relationship doubts can give rise to repeated discussions about your relationship's "rightness," which can be confusing and hurtful to a partner who doesn't understand your OCD. Finally, oversharing your obsessional thoughts can be alarming for a partner who might not understand that these intrusions don't reflect your true desires.

How has OCD interfered in *your* intimate relationships? This subject may not be fun to think about, but again, knowing what you're dealing with opens the door to solutions, like the ones offered later in this chapter. First, let's take a look at some common myths that can become problematic for romantic relationships when OCD is in the mix.

Separating Myths from Reality

There are a number of myths and misunderstandings about sexuality and other relationship dynamics that can make your relationship particularly susceptible to the effects of OCD. These myths all share the idea that life should fit into strict categories or be perfect in some way, which just isn't true. They create pressure to have everything figured out—whether it's your sexual orientation or standards that you set for yourself and your relationship—leading to compulsive overanalyzing. In reality, it's normal to have thoughts, feelings, or experiences that don't make sense or fit neatly into predefined categories. Trying to force everything into a perfect box only makes OCD worse by increasing anxiety and doubt. Correcting these misconceptions is important if they are contributing to your obsessions and compulsions. This foundational knowledge is also key to effectively applying the strategies that follow in this chapter.

Myth 1: Physical Responses "Down There" Reflect Your True Feelings

No matter your gender, intrusive unwanted thoughts involving sex can trigger physical sensations or changes in the genital region—a slight tingle, movement, or sense of swelling to more pronounced reactions like an erection or lubrication. This experience (sometimes called a "groinal response") is partly due to how our bodies are wired: The entire surface of our skin constantly sends sensory information to the brain. The genitals are especially packed with nerve endings, making them particularly sensitive. What's more, similar to sexual arousal, during moments of anxiety and fear (that is, the fight-or-flight response) your heart fiercely pumps blood all over your body, which is the reason you may notice increased sensations or activity "down there" when you become anxious. So, when your obsessional fear fixates on sexual topics like pedophilia, infidelity, or doubts about your sexual orientation, you might ironically experience signs of physical arousal and misinterpret them as confirming that your fears are coming true. This experience may add to your obsessional fear, creating a vicious cycle of obsessions, arousal sensations, misinterpretations, more obsessional fear, arousal, and so on.

Yet this sequence is triggered by a myth: that our physical reactions always reflect our mental state or values. They don't! The reality is that our physical reactions often don't match our personal feelings. *Experiencing general physical arousal or specific genital sensations in response to something that doesn't interest you does not automatically signify sexual desire or interest.* We all sometimes experience signs of arousal in response to stimuli we find unappealing and a turnoff. You may also notice these responses if you pay lots of attention to your genital area (like compulsively "scanning" for unwanted sensations). This increased focus can strengthen neural pathways over time, just like how chefs develop a finer sense of taste through repeated practice. By constantly checking and focusing on these sensations, you become more perceptive of even minor changes, perpetuating and intensifying the cycle of obsessional fear and heightened sensitivity.

So don't let these benign signs of arousal trick you into fearing that you're a bad person or a pervert or that you harbor sexual attraction toward undesired people or objects, as this obsession can get you stuck in the OCD vicious cycle. Your personal values and conscious choices play a far more important role in determining what or who you genuinely desire or find appealing. In other words, your *genitals* don't tell you what (or whom) you want or like; *you* do!

Myth 2: Sexual Orientation Fits into Strict Categories—and You Have to Choose One

Although we traditionally think of people as fitting into strict categories of sexual orientation—such as gay, straight, or bisexual—research shows that this idea is overly simplistic and doesn't reflect the true complexity of human sexuality. In reality, each person's sexual orientation includes elements often associated with different categories. To put it another way, labels like gay and straight correspond only to your predominant or primary romantic, emotional, and sexual attraction, but there's always going to be "noise." Straight people, for example, experience occasional feelings of attraction to the same sex (and vice versa). This is true of people with and without OCD, but it's particularly significant if you obsess over your sexual orientation. Again, *thoughts, feelings, and body sensations that don't align with your personal values or usual sexual interests are a normal part of being human.*

In other words, trying to definitively (compulsively) determine your sexual orientation, like whether you're *strictly* gay or straight, is pointless. It will only lead to more obsessional doubting because you'll inevitably have some experiences that fall outside the bounds of any chosen label. These atypical experiences fuel more obsessive fears and cause you to fixate on every little thought, feeling, or body sensation that doesn't seem to align with your perceived orientation. This hyperfocus only intensifies doubts and anxiety, trapping you in a cycle of compulsive overanalysis. Understand that it's normal for your feelings and attractions to sometimes deviate from your orientation and from the strict labels and categories that society has created.

Myth 3: There Is Such a Thing as a "Perfect Partnership"

Especially if you grapple with ROCD, it's important to know that relationships are inherently imperfect. For instance, it's normal for anyone—even people in long-term commitments and marriages—to occasionally question their relationship or wish it were different. Such doubts don't necessarily signal a lack of love or compatibility. Everyone has a mix of positive traits and imperfections, and it's only natural to sometimes notice and even feel annoyed by certain qualities or behaviors that you don't favor in your partner. Occasionally wanting (or fantasizing about) a partner with different physical or personality attributes is a common, natural experience.

If these normal relationship dynamics trigger anxiety and obsessive thoughts for you, remember that the concept of a "perfect" relationship, where you're always happy and intensely attracted to your partner, is a myth. Such relationships don't exist. What's more, expecting things to be perfect can lead to overanalyzing your relationship, getting stuck on senseless obsessional doubts, and missing out on the bigger picture and true joys of being with your partner. Recognizing that doubts and flaws are normal, and not a sign of deep personal or relationship problems, is important in managing ROCD and enjoying a more satisfying (and perfectly imperfect) partnership.

Myth 4: Honesty Means 100% Candor

It's important to be open and honest with your partner about significant issues that affect your relationship. But being open doesn't mean compulsively confessing your obsessive thoughts, particularly those that might upset your partner. Remember that obsessions do not reflect who you are as a person. Therefore, even if they focus on taboo topics, such as thinking of someone else, having ideas of being unfaithful, or the like, it's important to balance openness with discretion. Some privacy and personal boundaries are important ingredients in a healthy relationship. Choosing not to share your obsessions and other stray thoughts, feelings, and physical responses—especially if they might upset your partner and needlessly harm your relationship—is not a sign of dishonesty, betrayal, or deceit. Rather, this kind of privacy helps foster mutual respect and understanding between you and your partner; and it helps you manage OCD in a more constructive way.

Practical Tips for Managing OCD Symptoms in Your Relationship

The techniques from Chapters 3 and 4 can be applied to the knowledge you just gained to keep OCD symptoms from disrupting dating, emotional closeness, and physical intimacy. Below are some suggestions.

Achieving Physical Closeness Despite Contamination Fears

You can use many of the strategies from Chapter 3 to manage contamination obsessions in a relationship context. For example, if you're afraid of sexually transmitted infections (or other illnesses), write down your OCD story and ask yourself questions like "What would it take to be convinced that this story is realistic?" and "What concrete evidence do I have that either of us actually has an infection?" You could also try the life savings wager: Would you bet everything you own on the validity of your obsession? If not, why not?

If thoughts about germs show up during physical contact, the best tactic is to figuratively "drop the rope" instead of struggling with the obsession. Try tagging the thought or giving it a name to help you change your perspective; for example, "Oh, it's my old pal 'Dusty' reminding me that germs could be anywhere." These strategies allow you to maintain the closeness of the moment without interruption, even if the obsessional thought remains.

The ritual delay and modification strategies described in Chapter 4 are the best approaches for resisting urges to wash or clean or for asking your partner to do the same—especially if these urges surface during times of physical or emotional closeness. If your partner is aware of your OCD, you could arrange to have them hold you accountable, maybe by rewarding you for "surfing the compulsive urge" rather than by giving in and engaging in decontamination rituals.

Keeping Repugnant Thoughts from Taking Over Quality Time

When obsessions of a sexual, violent, or otherwise unwelcome nature come to mind during an intimate moment, your initial instinct is to fight them off as quickly as possible. Not only is this strategy ineffective, but it also diverts your attention away from your partner. The trick to staying in the moment is adopting a mind-set of awareness and acceptance. Instead of struggling with obsessive thoughts, consider them background mental noise rather than *facts*. If the image of a child or family member pops into your mind during sex, make room for it as if it's tagging along for the ride. I know that this suggestion seems odd, but taking this kind of nonjudgmental stance toward your thoughts will enable you to remain in the present moment compared to the effort spent resisting these mental intrusions. Remember that *what you resist persists,* but allowing thoughts to come and go freely helps reduce their power over you and allows you to focus on what truly matters.

Feeling Confident in Spite of ROCD

Taking negative thoughts about your relationship at face value will only intensify your obsessional fear. But there's another way to look at ROCD obsessions: They're actually a reflection of how much you value your relationship. These thoughts only seem threatening because they challenge something you deeply care about. In other words, if your partner and your relationship weren't important to you, these obsessive thoughts wouldn't have such an impact. Your distress over these thoughts indicates a strong emotional investment in the relationship. It's the significance of your relationship and your commitment to your partner that make these obsessions so potent, not necessarily the truth or likelihood of the thoughts themselves. Essentially, your distress is proportional to the value you place on your relationship.

Although many of the strategies in Chapter 3 can be applied to relationship obsessions, discrediting them is a good place to start. Write down the reasons you doubt your love for your partner or the "rightness" of your relationship. Then develop your OCD story and look carefully at the basis for your worries. Are your worries grounded in common sense and concrete facts, or are they more a product of your imagination, faulty reasoning, and hypothetical possibilities? There's probably little or no solid evidence to back up your obsessive fears, and neither do your intentions and judgment provide any real validation. You can also challenge your ROCD symptoms with a reality check:

Ask yourself what tangible evidence and rational arguments you would need from someone else to convince you that *their* relationship was wrong or that *their* love isn't genuine. When you compare this information to the reasons *you* buy into *your* obsessional doubts, does your perspective change?

Moving beyond Guilt and Confession Rituals

As discussed earlier, it's important to balance honesty with privacy regarding your obsessions. If you experience guilt and the urge to confess unwanted intrusive thoughts to your partner, here's how you can apply the strategies from Chapters 3 and 4 to manage these obsessions and resist compulsive urges.

First, remember that the distress caused by these thoughts is a testament to your strong moral compass. In other words, the reason these thoughts disturb you is that your ethical standards are so stringent that you consider even having such thoughts to be out of bounds. Your high standards are a clear sign of your integrity and dedication to your partner. Keep this fact in mind when you use the strategies in Chapter 3 for discrediting your obsessions. Look for examples of inferential confusion and practice recognizing the differences between the imagined feared self in your OCD story and what the concrete evidence and your common sense are telling you.

Second, remember that having unwanted obsessional thoughts is fundamentally different from actually cheating or acting dishonestly or deceitfully. Obsessions are involuntary. You can't prevent them, and they do not reflect your true character, values, or intentions. On the other hand, actual wrongdoing involves a conscious decision. Also, thoughts do not directly affect others or violate laws or ethics. Imagine if the legal system held people accountable for their *thoughts* of wrongdoing (we'd all be in jail!). Finally, as echoed throughout this book, the human brain generates thousands of thoughts each day, including undesirable or uncomfortable ones. Your ability to think about doing something wrong and then choose not to do it is a sign of ethical self-reflection, good moral judgment, and your commitment to your relationship and your values. You don't need to listen when OCD taunts you otherwise.

Working Together to Build an OCD-Resilient Relationship

If you're in a long-term relationship, it's beneficial to complement the strategies outlined in the previous section by collaborating with your partner. This joint effort will help minimize the impact of OCD on your relationship and strengthen your closeness and intimacy. I recommend reading and discussing the material in this section together as a powerful step toward a healthier partnership in which you're both actively addressing the challenges posed by OCD in a constructive way. I also suggest sitting down together and carefully reviewing (and practicing) the productive communication strategies introduced in Chapter 8. The better you're able to share thoughts and feelings, actively listen, and work together to make decisions, the less anxiety and conflict you'll encounter.

Recognizing Accommodation in Your Relationship

Chapter 8 introduced the idea of accommodation, in which other people modify their routines or take on extra duties to help you manage your OCD symptoms. In intimate relationships, accommodation can manifest in various ways:

- Your partner takes on tasks that could trigger your obsessions, such as opening doors for you if you have a fear of germs from doorknobs or doing all the driving if you're worried about causing an accident.

- Together, you and your partner steer clear of scenarios that might activate your OCD, such as choosing not to go to the state fair because of concerns about contamination from large groups of people.

- Your partner participates in rituals, such as by helping you check that doors are locked or by listening to your repeated confessions of intrusive thoughts.

Whether your partner willingly accommodates your OCD as an expression of care and concern or does so reluctantly to prevent conflicts, the purpose of accommodation is to provide you with comfort. But this is not an effective long-term solution—the obsessions and anxiety eventually resurface, leading to the need for more and more accommodation and resulting in frustration. Accommodation can also become so deeply integrated into your relationship that it becomes invisible to you and your partner.

To address accommodation you need to be able to recognize when it's happening. The table on page 142 provides examples of how accommodation can occur. Start by reviewing these examples with your partner and discuss any patterns that seem familiar in your relationship.

Sharing Pleasant Activities

For some couples, accommodation becomes an important way of saying "I care about you" or "I love you." But while love, support, and connection are important in your relationship, it's not healthy if they revolve predominantly around OCD. For your relationship to flourish, the closeness you experience should come from jointly engaging in activities that both of you equally enjoy. So, next discuss ways you can enjoy each other's company and feel connected outside of OCD's grasp and focus on activities that are not primarily about reducing anxiety. If you need inspiration, consult the list of suggestions on page 143. Then, using decision-making skills, commit to incorporating one or more of these activities into your weekly routine, creating moments you both can look forward to and enjoy together.

Reducing Accommodation Together

Once you've begun sharing enjoyable activities together, you're ready to work as a team to reduce accommodation. Beginning on page 143 are six steps to guide you through this process, ensuring clear communication, mutual understanding, respect, and support. The goal is to achieve a dynamic in which you acknowledge OCD but don't let it overshadow your emotional or physical connection.

How Accommodation Happens: Helping with Avoidance

Your partner changes their routine for you.	You avoid together as a couple.
Nick works in a hospital, but his partner, Samantha, is afraid of germs. So Nick changes out of his work clothes before entering the house.	Emily has obsessional fears about food poisoning. Consequently, she and her partner, Joe, avoid eating at restaurants.
Heidi doesn't want Josh to experience anxiety and doubt about his salvation, so she avoids talking about religion, even though she is a devout Christian.	Paul now sleeps in a separate room (even though he would prefer to sleep with Liam) because Liam has obsessions that he will impulsively act on unwanted obsessional thoughts of harming Paul in his sleep.
Because Anika has obsessions of losing control and molesting the baby, Rohan has taken over responsibilities such as changing all of the diapers and giving all of the baths.	Justine obsesses that the number 13 will bring "bad luck." On the last trip she and Chris took together, the hotel gave them room 13. When they learned that all the other rooms were taken, they decided to go to a different hotel.

How Accommodation Happens: Helping with Rituals

Your partner participates in rituals.	Your partner provides reassurance.
Talia has obsessions about fires and break-ins, so she insists that Ariel help with nightly checking rituals of all appliances, windows, and doors. Ariel even takes pictures to reassure Talia that everything is off or locked.	Nina obsesses that she might have said something insulting in a text or social media post, so she and Ira sit down and review each of her texts and posts, with Ira reassuring her that they're not offensive.
Leigh listens to Marty's compulsive confession of the "sins" that he is afraid he has committed each day.	When Jacques obsesses that he might have hit a pedestrian with his car, Martine comforts him and assures him he would definitely be aware if such an incident had occurred.
After 10 years of marriage, Joel knows when to wash his hands and take extra showers to keep Kylie from becoming anxious. He willingly completes these rituals without Kylie having to request it.	Maria obsesses that she has been unfaithful to Tyrone and often asks him for reassurance that she is not an adulterer for noticing other attractive men or thinking about old boyfriends. Tyrone knows just what to say to calm her fears.

Joint Activities for Couples

- Going to a concert
- Attending a lecture
- Going to a sporting event
- Having a picnic
- Hiking
- Preparing a special meal
- Taking photographs
- Going dancing
- Jogging or working out
- Staying overnight at a hotel
- Listening to music
- Shopping
- Working in the garden/mowing the lawn
- Going to a museum or zoo
- Visiting friends or relatives
- Making a photo album
- Volunteering in the community
- Having breakfast in bed
- Taking a walk
- Going to a movie or show
- Going out for dinner
- Biking
- Playing golf or tennis
- Playing board games
- Going bowling
- Working on a joint hobby
- Taking a class together
- Going to a park
- Camping out
- Playing musical instruments
- Going out for dessert
- Playing video games
- Working on a household project
- Studying the family genealogy
- Bird watching or star gazing
- Going out for a drive
- Giving each other a massage

STEP 1: IDENTIFY A TARGET

Choose one accommodation behavior you both agree to address. This could be anything from assisting less with washing or checking rituals to not providing reassurance about certain fears. It's okay to start small so you're likely to have success.

STEP 2: DEVELOP A PLAN

Create a plan that lays out exactly what actions each of you will take. For example, *you* will refrain from confessing certain unwanted thoughts or asking for reassurance about a particular topic, and *your partner* will refrain from listening to confessions, answering questions, performing particular rituals, or the like. Importantly, your partner should also give you plenty of praise and support (see Step 3).

STEP 3: PUT THE PLAN INTO ACTION

Now implement your plan, but do it gradually. Use the strategies proposed earlier in this chapter (and those in Chapters 3 and 4) to help manage obsessional thoughts, anxiety, and compulsive urges as you adjust to the changes in accommodation. Your partner can help you cope with anxiety by offering words of support and encouragement rather than stepping in to eliminate the anxiety for you. Below are some supportive statements your partner can use. Notice they are not designed to give you reassurance but to help you get through the temporary distress.

- I know this is hard and I have faith in you—you can get through this!
- I'm here with you. You're not alone in this.
- You are strong and resilient—you've got this!
- I love you, and I know how strong you are.
- Think about the pride you'll feel once you've overcome this.
- You've overcome challenges before, and I know you can do it this time.
- I'm so proud of you for giving it a try.

STEP 4: MONITOR, ADJUST, AND CELEBRATE PROGRESS

Have regular discussions in which you share thoughts and feelings about how the process is going. Are adjustments needed? Is the pace comfortable for you both? Be flexible and modify your plan as needed using decision-making skills. Think of it as a team effort—both of you should feel heard and supported throughout the process. And be sure to recognize and celebrate the progress you make, no matter how small, which helps in building confidence and motivation to continue.

STEP 5: EXPAND YOUR FOCUS

After successfully decreasing accommodation in one area, move ahead and tackle it in another, and another, and so on. View this process not just as a means to reduce accommodation, but also as an opportunity to fortify your relationship through teamwork, mutual understanding, support, and encouragement.

STEP 6: CONSIDER HEALTHY SUPPORT ACTIVITIES

If you and your partner are open to it, attend a support group together to enhance your partner's understanding of OCD and your own experiences with it. If you're receiving treatment, think about talking to your therapist about having your partner join one or more sessions. This kind of support could provide your partner with a better understanding of the therapy process.

Strategies for Resolving Conflicts and Navigating Breakups

From misunderstandings about OCD symptoms to the stress of accommodating the disorder, conflicts can arise and strain your relationships. Managing disagreements requires effective communication to understand each other's perspective. The tips in the next sections can be helpful in resolving conflicts and coping with relationship breakups against the backdrop of OCD.

Understanding and Managing Conflict

There are various sources of relationship conflict related to OCD. Most commonly, disagreements stem from OCD-related disruption of activities, emotional stress, financial pressures, social limitations, and changes in roles within the relationship. For example, your partner might feel annoyed by having to adjust their routine or take on extra responsibilities to accommodate OCD. But conflict can also arise from misunderstandings in which your partner doesn't grasp the nature of your symptoms, resulting in misconceptions about your behaviors. For example, your partner might misinterpret your reassurance-seeking rituals as a sign that you don't trust them. Differences in expectations regarding support may also lead to conflict; for instance, if your partner is reluctant to join you in therapy sessions despite your desire for their involvement.

Resolving conflict begins with sharing thoughts and feelings and practicing active listening. For example, if you are upset because your partner refuses to attend a support group with you, try to understand their position (even if you disagree) and express your perspective calmly, rather than immediately resorting to anger or making accusatory statements, which will further escalate the conflict. Once you understand one another, shift to decision-making strategies to seek a compromise—a middle ground that considers your needs and those of your partner. If conflicts become particularly challenging, consider involving a mediator, such as a mental health professional, who can provide an objective viewpoint and guide you toward solutions that respect everyone's needs.

Recovering from a Breakup

Experiencing a breakup can intensify OCD symptoms and may lead to a compulsive overanalysis of the relationship and ruminating about where things went wrong and what could have been done differently. So be ready to use the techniques discussed in Chapters 3 and 4 for managing obsessions and compulsions. OCD flourishes in turbulent environments, so if you're still in contact with your ex-partner, establish clear boundaries, as outlined in Chapter 6, and consider reducing your interactions for a while. Distancing yourself will help minimize additional stress, allowing you to prioritize your own mental health and well-being.

It's also helpful to stick to a structured schedule and maintain your daily routine. The sense of control can be reassuring. Make sure to eat regular meals, get adequate sleep, and set aside time for exercise and relaxation. If you enjoy mindfulness practices such as meditation or yoga, now is the time to lean into these activities to reduce anxiety and increase moments of peace and clarity. Engaging in hobbies or interests can also serve as a buffer against the stress and anxiety that are common companions of both OCD and relationship endings. These activities not only offer a diversion from obsessional thoughts, but also foster your sense of self and personal fulfillment during a time when you might feel especially vulnerable.

Most important, lean on your support network. Reach out to friends or family who are understanding. Their emotional support and insights are incredibly valuable. Consider engaging with a therapist who is adept at navigating the emotional intricacies of a breakup. A professional with expertise in OCD can provide you with customized advice and coping mechanisms. Joining an OCD support group can also be helpful during a breakup since such groups offer a platform to exchange similar experiences, providing comfort and a feeling of community and mutual understanding.

The strategies described in this chapter can empower you to build and maintain fulfilling close relationships, despite the hurdles OCD might place in your path. Remember, understanding yourself and effectively communicating with your partner are key to fostering a resilient and supportive partnership. The next chapter addresses another critical aspect of living well: how to keep OCD from holding you back from achieving your academic and professional goals.

Practical Steps for Living Well: Thriving in Romantic Relationships

Be open about OCD:

- Discuss how OCD affects you and your relationship, whether it is new or long term.
- Encourage your partner to learn about OCD to better understand and support you.

Practice communication skills:

- Use the sharing thoughts and feelings and active listening skills from Chapter 8 when discussing OCD.
- Set boundaries regarding when and how much to discuss OCD to prevent it from dominating your relationship.

Address OCD symptoms that impact your relationship:

- Use strategies from Chapters 3 and 4 to tackle obsessions and compulsions that interfere with intimacy.
- Set limits on reassurance seeking with the help of your partner.

Engage in joint activities:

- Have fun together to strengthen your connection outside of OCD.
- Schedule regular date nights or special outings to prioritize quality time together.

Reduce accommodation together:

- Identify and discuss accommodation behaviors in your relationship.
- Develop a plan to reduce accommodation, with mutual support and encouragement.

10

navigating work and school

As you know, OCD can complicate the completion of tasks in different ways. Unwanted thoughts may intrude on the mental processes that allow you to write a report or an essay, solve a problem at work, or design a new product. Compulsive rituals may take up time you need to meet a deadline. Questions about how much to disclose about your OCD can make communications with bosses, coworkers, teachers, and classmates challenging. This chapter focuses on how to keep OCD from derailing your productivity during work hours or within the halls of education. Besides providing self-help tactics for living well in these important domains of life, the chapter guides you through modifications to your work or school environment that can ease the challenges posed by obsessions and compulsions and facilitate more effective functioning.

How Does OCD Interfere at Work or in the Classroom?

Do you feel like you're always playing catch-up or being overwhelmed by your workload? Do these examples sound familiar?

- Elliott, a college student, has a compulsion to read every line of his textbooks multiple times to ensure he hasn't missed anything. This ritual cuts into his study time and ability to complete assignments on schedule.

- When Maku's obsessional thoughts about sex or blasphemy show up, she has the compulsive urge to repeat whatever she's doing at the time. This compulsion gets in the way of taking notes in class, writing papers, and answering exam questions.

- Ryan's need for perfect alignment in his designs causes his firm to miss deadlines for proposals and creates a backlog of work.

- Anna obsesses that she mistakenly used insensitive language in her emails to work colleagues. She gets stuck checking and revising her messages over and over before finally sending them.

- Diego's OCD manifests in a compulsion to check and recheck his code for errors, which slows down his work, affecting project timelines and his ability to meet deadlines.

- Rachel, a high school teacher, has an obsessional fear of cold sores. She spends excessive time sanitizing her classroom and even avoids certain students. These symptoms impact her lesson preparation and ability to engage with other people.

To gain a deeper understanding of how OCD affects your work or school life, try this reflective journaling activity: Each day, for two to three weeks, dedicate some time to writing down instances when OCD influenced your productivity, interactions, or emotions at work or school. Describe the situation, the OCD symptoms you experienced, and their impact on your tasks or interactions. Then review your entries to identify patterns. What are the common triggers or times when symptoms intensify? How did OCD affect your relationships with colleagues or peers and your ability to meet deadlines or complete tasks? The strategies in this chapter will assist you in developing coping strategies and accommodation requests tailored to these identified patterns, enhancing your ability to manage OCD effectively in both professional and educational environments.

Strategies for Managing OCD at Work and School

You can adapt most of the strategies discussed throughout this book to manage OCD symptoms in your work or study environment. However, the following methods are tailored specifically to minimize the influence of obsessional fears and compulsive behaviors in your professional and academic pursuits.

Keep a Consistent Routine

Remember, OCD thrives in turbulence. Adhering to a regular daily routine creates a predictable environment, which reduces the uncertainty that can intensify anxiety and OCD. If you don't already have one, consider creating a structured daily plan that specifies times for waking up, attending work or school, eating meals, taking breaks, relaxing, and any other daily activities. Commit to following this schedule for a fixed period, like two weeks, and take time each day to reflect on how well you stuck to this routine and the obstacles you encountered. After each week, go over these reflections to spot any recurring patterns and adjust your schedule accordingly.

At the same time, remember the importance of flexibility. Work and school (and life in general) have their own set of variable demands, and being able to adapt your routine to these changes is crucial. This balance ensures that your routine is both realistic and sustainable long term. By maintaining a schedule that is both structured and adaptable, you create a supportive environment for managing OCD, enhancing your functionality and well-being.

Divide Up Complex Tasks and Projects

If you find yourself overwhelmed by complicated or daunting tasks, such as work projects or term papers, try thinking about them as smaller, more manageable steps. Begin by listing all the steps required to accomplish the task. Next, approach this work in stages, like researching the topic, organizing your notes, and writing individual sections. Then arrange these tasks in a practical order that reflects the logical progression of the overall project and focus on completing them one at a time. For instance, start with foundational tasks such as gathering research materials and understanding the topic, followed by developing a structured outline. Proceed with writing the introduction, then work through the various sections one at a time. Concentrating on one stage at a time helps maintain your focus, reducing anxiety and making the entire process more approachable and less daunting.

Prioritize Effectively

If OCD slows down your productivity, concentrate on tasks of the highest importance to ensure that your energy is invested wisely. Begin by assessing all your tasks, identifying the most crucial ones, taking into account their importance and the implications of not completing them promptly. Focus primarily on these responsibilities. Keep in mind that not all tasks can be equally urgent and that recognizing the most critical ones helps you channel your efforts more effectively. Also, dedicate your peak productivity hours to these high-priority tasks, choosing times when you're most alert and least impacted by OCD symptoms.

Stay Organized

Countless organizational tools can help you keep track of deadlines and structure your day. If you don't already use one, consider starting now. Such tools significantly minimize the chaos and uncertainty that often trigger or exacerbate OCD symptoms, providing a sense of control and clarity. Planners and calendars allow you to visually map out your responsibilities, appointments, and deadlines, making it easier to see what needs to be done and when. A visual representation of your schedule can be reassuring, reducing the anxiety associated with forgetting or overlooking important tasks. If writing your to-do list on paper helps solidify it in your mind, you might prefer a physical planner. On the other hand, digital calendars have the advantage of being easily editable and accessible from multiple devices. Some smartphone apps offer features like reminders, due-date notifications, and the ability to categorize tasks into different projects or classes. Some even allow you to separate tasks into subtasks, making larger projects feel more manageable. Look for apps that sync across all your devices, ensuring that you have access to your organizational system whether you're at home, work, or school.

Also consider setting up a designated workspace where you can keep all your work or study materials organized. This setup could involve organizing your digital files into specific folders on your computer, keeping your desk clutter free, or having a specific place to store all your study materials. A well-organized workspace reduces distractions and makes it easier to focus on the task at hand.

The goal of using these organizational tools is to create and maintain a structured and predictable environment. By keeping track of your responsibilities and structuring your day, you can reduce the anxiety and stress that accompany OCD, allowing you to focus more on your work or studies. Experiment with different tools and setups to find what works best for you and be open to adjusting your system as your needs change.

Keep Daily Stress in Check

Maintaining control over daily stress is crucial when managing OCD in professional and academic settings. Helpful strategies include practicing mindfulness and relaxation techniques, like deep breathing exercises, which can be integrated into your daily routine to refocus and ground yourself during overwhelming moments. Regular breaks throughout the day are also essential, allowing time for relaxing and resetting your focus.

Staying physically active is another effective method to clear your mind and improve concentration. Simple exercises like a brisk walk around the office or campus can significantly lower anxiety levels and boost mental clarity. Additionally, optimizing your work or study environment to minimize distractions and create a comfortable space can enhance concentration. Finally, practicing self-compassion and acknowledging your daily achievements, no matter how small, instills a positive mind-set. This approach helps not only in coping with OCD, but also in enhancing overall performance and resilience in your professional and academic life.

Understanding and Exercising Your Legal Rights to Accommodations

While self-guided strategies can be a big help, they may not always be sufficient in highly demanding or competitive environments like work or school. In these settings, securing specific *accommodations* might be the key to unlocking your full potential and really thriving. In academic and employment spheres, accommodations are official procedural modifications or adjustments to support people with disabilities or specific needs, ensuring that they have equal access and opportunities. (It's important to distinguish between this *helpful* type of accommodation and the *unhelpful* type of family accommodation mentioned in Chapter 8. Work or school accommodations are formally authorized supportive changes aimed at fostering your success. Family accommodations involve others' changing their routine or taking on added responsibilities in an effort to minimize your distress in the moment, but in a way that only makes OCD worse in the long term.) The list on the facing page shows examples of common work- and school-based accommodations for people with OCD.

Fortunately, established resources and procedures are available to help you obtain these necessary modifications.

What Are Your Rights under the Law?

Certain laws safeguard the rights of people with psychological disorders such as OCD. These regulations mandate that workplaces and educational institutions make or provide reasonable accommodations, ensuring that you have equal access to employment and education opportunities.

Common Work and School Accommodations for People with OCD

- Quiet workspaces to improve concentration
- Short breaks to perform rituals or manage stress
- The option to work or learn from home to manage OCD symptoms
- Flexibility with deadlines (or extra time for exams) when OCD symptoms become disruptive
- Part-time work options if the full workload exacerbates OCD symptoms
- Assistance in managing communication-related tasks
- Detailed instructions for tasks to reduce anxiety associated with uncertainty or mistakes
- Access to counseling or support services or on-site mental health services

THE AMERICANS WITH DISABILITIES ACT (ADA)

The ADA is a U.S. law protecting the rights of people with disabilities. It prevents discrimination in public areas such as employment, education, and transportation. The ADA defines a disability as an impairment that significantly restricts major life activities. Since OCD qualifies as a disability, employers are obligated to offer reasonable accommodations, provided they don't impose undue hardship on the business.

SECTION 504 OF THE REHABILITATION ACT OF 1973

This law protects the rights of people with disabilities in programs and activities that receive federal financial assistance, including schools. Under Section 504, students with disabilities, including those with OCD, have the right to receive accommodations and modifications to ensure equal access to education.

INDIVIDUALS WITH DISABILITIES EDUCATION ACT (IDEA)

This law applies to public elementary, middle, and high schools. Although IDEA primarily focuses on students with learning disabilities, it can also apply to students with other disabilities that affect their educational performance, including OCD.

How to Pursue Workplace Accommodations

To request accommodations at work you'll need to disclose that you have OCD and provide written documentation to verify that you qualify for accommodations. As discussed in Chapter 6, this decision should be made with a thorough understanding of the benefits and risks. Evaluate your work environment and its culture—is it supportive and understanding of mental health issues? Disclosure, along with providing documentation, is necessary to receive support and accommodations, but it also carries risks like potential stigma or altered perceptions from colleagues. If your workplace seems understanding, it's probably worth opening up about your OCD so you can gain accommodations. If you're uncertain, seek advice from someone in your support network or a professional.

Before raising the topic of accommodations with your boss or supervisor, you'll want to make sure you're prepared to clearly articulate your needs. Start by identifying particular modifications or support that could assist you in better managing OCD in the workplace. Then think about how these accommodations would enhance your performance. Write down these details to give you confidence and help you effectively convey your needs. For example:

- A more flexible start time would help me be more focused when I get to work.
- Extended deadlines would help me complete my work with less anxiety.
- The option to work from home would minimize disruption from my washing rituals.

Remember: It's your right to seek accommodations. So when the moment comes to make a formal request, approach the conversation with confidence and self-assertion. Depending on your particular workplace, reach out to a direct supervisor or the human resources (HR) department. You'll likely need to present documentation from a health care provider confirming your OCD diagnosis, as well as details of how your symptoms impact job performance. Be ready to provide clear, concrete examples of how OCD affects your job duties and how the proposed accommodations can ease these challenges and boost your productivity. For instance, you might explain: "I find that my concentration is significantly impacted by intrusive thoughts, and having the flexibility to work in a quieter space would help me focus better." Here's how you might take the previous examples and turn them into requests:

- "I sometimes get stuck doing rituals in the morning that can make me late. A flexible start time would reduce my stress and make me more focused when I arrive."

- "Because of my need to repeatedly check things, it takes me longer to complete tasks. If I could have extended deadlines, I would be able to complete my work with less anxiety and more thoroughness."

- "I have a compulsion to wash my hands frequently, which can be disruptive in an office setting. Having the ability to work from home when I'm having difficulty with these rituals would greatly reduce this disruption."

Make sure to emphasize that these accommodations will not just benefit *you* but also boost overall workplace productivity. For example, "By being able to work from home, I can do my washing rituals without disrupting everyone else when I'm constantly getting up to go to the sink." The goal is to promote an understanding of your needs and how addressing them can lead to a more positive outcome for both you and your employer.

Be open-minded and prepared to compromise if your initial requests aren't feasible for one reason or another. Use the communication skills described in Chapter 8 and be open to negotiating the extent or duration of accommodations, perhaps suggesting a trial period to assess their effectiveness. Your willingness to find mutually beneficial solutions that don't impose undue burdens on your employer can significantly increase the chances of reaching a satisfactory agreement. Conversely, displaying excessive arrogance or entitlement or making unreasonable demands can hinder your chances of obtaining what you need.

Finally, be sure to keep a written record of all interactions and agreements related to your request for accommodations, including your proposals and your employer's responses. This record provides a basis for accountability and ensures that both parties adhere to the agreed terms. Such records also serve as a reference for any future discussions or adjustments to the accommodations and offer legal protection by demonstrating that you have followed proper procedures and communicated your needs clearly.

How to Request Accommodations in School

To obtain accommodations that would support your academic performance, begin by acquiring a formal diagnosis of OCD from a mental health professional. This should be accompanied by a detailed report from your clinician that outlines how the disorder impacts educational activities, including studying, concentration, class attendance, and taking exams. The report should also recommend specific academic accommodations that would be beneficial.

Next schedule a meeting with your school's Accessibility Resources and Services (ARS) Office, a step *you* need to initiate. This office ensures that students with disabilities receive necessary supports, aligned with legal and institutional standards. In this confidential meeting, discuss your OCD challenges and suggest accommodations like extra test time, a quiet exam space, note-taking assistance, or flexible deadlines. The ARS office will assess your needs against ADA and Section 504 criteria to confirm eligibility, then collaborate with you to develop a customized accommodation plan. Typically, the ARS office provides a letter to your instructors outlining the plan without disclosing your diagnosis. However, I recommend directly checking with your instructors to reassure yourself that they are prepared to provide the required support. If your situation changes or the accommodations aren't meeting your needs, promptly communicate this information to your professors and the ARS office so that suitable changes can be made.

Keep in mind that the process may differ slightly based on your educational institution and personal circumstances. The cornerstone of successfully acquiring accommodations is maintaining open communication and actively engaging with your college's disability services.

What to Expect from the Process

CONFIDENTIALITY

Confidentiality ensures that your privacy is protected and that the details of your OCD are disclosed only to people directly involved in facilitating your accommodations, which may include certain personnel in HR, supervisors, or school ARS staff. Moreover, the information shared is limited to what is absolutely necessary to implement the accommodations. Conversations regarding your needs are conducted discreetly to maintain a respectful and comfortable environment. While it's important to recognize that certain people may need to be informed to effectively provide accommodations, they are also obligated to maintain confidentiality. This approach both safeguards your personal information and creates a supportive atmosphere, allowing you to focus on your professional or academic responsibilities without the added concern of privacy issues.

A SWIFT RESPONSE

Employers and educational institutions are expected to respond promptly to accommodation requests, although the actual time frame can vary depending on factors such as the complexity of your request and organizational procedures. This prompt response is mandated under the ADA to avoid causing you unnecessary difficulties. While delays can occur due to administrative reasons or the need for additional information, you are entitled to ongoing communication about the status of your request and an estimated response time.

QUESTIONS FROM COLLEAGUES OR PEERS

If you decide to disclose your OCD, be ready to inform others about your accommodations while establishing clear boundaries about what you're willing to discuss. When responding to questions, aim to be brief and focus on how you handle your OCD at work or school. As discussed in Chapter 6, feel free to express discomfort in answering specific queries. And if interactions with colleagues or peers become difficult, remember that you can always seek assistance from a supervisor,

HR representative, or a counselor. Doing so balances openness with personal comfort and ensures you have access to support when needed.

Long-Term Strategies for Success

Succeeding in professional or academic environments while dealing with OCD involves more than just daily coping; it requires strategizing for long-term success. The following tactics can help you establish a lasting trajectory toward achievement, balancing OCD management with your career and educational aspirations.

Create a Personal Action Plan

Developing an action plan that's tailored to your specific needs and circumstances can further help you handle your symptoms and achieve your goals. Start by setting clear, attainable objectives for yourself. Here are some examples:

- Improve my ability to manage time effectively
- Increase my capacity to stay focused on certain tasks
- Enhance my coping skills to better handle stressful situations at work or school
- Complete a challenging course with good grades
- Get a desired promotion at work
- Build stronger relationships with colleagues, peers, or mentors

Next reflect on the strategies and coping mechanisms that have worked for you in the past—therapy skills, relaxation techniques, or daily routines that help manage your symptoms. Work to integrate them into your regular schedule to provide consistency in your approach to managing OCD.

Regularly review and adjust your action plan. OCD symptoms can fluctuate, and life circumstances change. As a result, the strategies that once worked may need to be modified or replaced. Periodic reviews allow you to stay responsive to these changes and ensure that your approach remains effective and relevant.

Consider incorporating professional guidance into your action plan. Working with a therapist or counselor can help you refine your strategies so that they align with both your personal and professional or academic goals. A mental health professional can offer new insights, support, and accountability, helping you navigate the challenges of OCD with more confidence and effectiveness.

Stay Informed

In addition to remaining up-to-date on the latest developments in OCD treatment and research, be sure to keep up with any changes to the law and how it relates to your rights in the workplace or educational settings. Read reputable articles and studies that provide well-researched, current information from credible sources. Attend workshops and participate in webinars. Engaging with the OCD community, whether through support groups or online forums, opens doors to a wealth of shared experiences and insights. These interactions can be incredibly valuable, offering new perspectives and strategies that you may not have considered. The support and understanding from others facing similar struggles can also be a significant source of emotional strength and encouragement.

As you accumulate knowledge and insights, consider educating those in your immediate environment. Sharing what you've learned with peers, colleagues, and educators can help create a more supportive and accommodating environment. It's not just about advocacy but also about fostering empathy and cooperation from those around you. The more people understand the challenges and nuances of OCD, the more they can help create a conducive atmosphere that acknowledges and respects your needs.

Celebrate Successes and Learn from Challenges

Taking pride in your accomplishments and learning from your challenges are important for living well with OCD in both your professional and academic environments. Recognizing and celebrating even the smallest achievements can have a significant impact on your morale and motivation. These achievements could range from effectively managing your symptoms during a particularly stressful period to meeting a specific goal at work or school. Celebrating these victories, no matter how small, reinforces positive behavior and boosts your confidence.

Reflecting on challenges is just as important. But instead of viewing difficulties as setbacks, consider them opportunities for learning and growth. Analyze what didn't work and why and think about how you can adjust your approach for a better outcome next time. This kind of reflective analysis after the fact is essential for evolving and enhancing your strategy in managing despite having OCD.

Finally, maintaining a positive outlook is essential. Focus on your strengths and the progress you've made so far. A positive mind-set not only enhances your ability to cope with OCD, but also fosters resilience and long-term success. It's a reminder that despite the challenges, you have the capacity to grow and thrive.

By developing a personalized action plan, staying informed, and adopting a balanced perspective on your successes and challenges, you lay a strong foundation for ongoing success. Remember, managing OCD is a continual journey, and you possess the strength and resources to navigate it successfully, whether in your professional or your academic life.

Practical Steps for Living Well: Navigating Work and School

Request accommodations:

- Understand your legal rights and the types of accommodations that can help you succeed.
- Clearly explain how accommodations will boost your academic or work productivity.
- Keep records of all communications about your requests.

Simplify and prioritize tasks:

- Divide large tasks into smaller steps.
- Create lists of high-, medium-, and low-importance tasks to invest energy where it matters.

Maintain a routine—with flexibility:

- Create a daily schedule with times to wake up, attend work/school, eat meals, take breaks, and relax.
- Build in flexibility to adapt to unexpected changes or demands.

Stay organized:

- Use a planner or digital app to track task progress and deadlines.
- Keep your desk clutter free and use folders to sort digital files.

11

surviving a crisis

A crisis is a sudden, intense event that significantly disrupts your life, creating acute stress and anxiety. Crises are particularly challenging when you have OCD because they often require quick decisions and swift actions, and therefore clash with the need for reassurance and certainty. Examples include medical emergencies, the sudden loss of a loved one, natural disasters, job loss, or academic setbacks. But crises can also occur if your obsessional fears are realized, such as direct exposure to (or actually contracting) the illness you've been obsessively worried about, learning that you actually *did* make the costly mistake you've been afraid of making, or facing public humiliation if you have obsessions about offending others. Crises not only pose immediate complications, obstacles, threats, and hardships; they can also trigger significant life changes that push your coping mechanisms to their limits.

This book has focused primarily on managing OCD symptoms as they affect your everyday life. Crises, fortunately, are not a daily occurrence for most people. But they are part of life. And when they come up, they pose unique challenges that call for a quick and decisive response. You may need to implement measures in addition to the strategies you've learned so far in this book. This chapter provides strategies for managing the intense and unpredictable period following a significant emergency, aiming to help you balance these dynamic changes with your need for control and certainty.

The Intersection of OCD and Crisis

A crisis results in mental shock often characterized by feelings of disbelief and confusion. You can feel knocked off balance by the unpredictability of life. It disrupts your routine and necessitates swift decisions. These rapid changes and looming uncertainties can be particularly destabilizing, disrupting your assurance that your world is predictable and you can exert some control over it. This loss of footing exacerbates obsessional fear and compulsions. For example, if you have contamination obsessions, you might find that washing and cleaning rituals increase during a health crisis like a pandemic. If you have an obsessional fear of harm or mistakes, you might have stronger urges to check appliances, alarms, or locks, even when it's not practical to do so. The need for reassurance is also likely to increase when faced with a crisis. For example, you might continually ask questions seeking certainty or spend lots of time mentally reviewing conversations to ensure you didn't say anything offensive.

These compulsions are your attempts to reduce fear and regain control or certainty. However, the escalation in OCD symptoms only complicates the situation. For instance, you might avoid necessary evacuations during a fire or natural disaster owing to fears of contamination outside of your controlled environment. Your ability to make critical decisions might be impaired by the overwhelming need to focus on completing mental reviewing rituals.

So a crisis doesn't merely add to daily challenges; it intricately interacts with OCD symptoms, creating a cycle in which the crisis exacerbates OCD symptoms, which in turn makes managing the crisis more daunting. This cycle highlights the need for customized strategies to effectively address both the external difficulties of the crisis and the internal challenges of OCD.

Crisis-Coping Strategies with OCD

A crisis can trigger a range of reactions, from feeling overwhelmed to experiencing full-on mental shock, which includes sudden numbness or disorientation, trouble processing thoughts or emotions, a feeling of being detached from reality, and physical signs such as shaking, a rapid heartbeat, or breathlessness. Chapters 3 and 4 provide a wealth of strategies and exercises for managing the intensification of obsessions and compulsions. The table below can remind you of several quick, in-the-moment tactics that work best to immediately manage obsessive fears or compulsions that intensify rapidly during a crisis. Throughout this chapter I'll describe how to apply these tactics in different types of situations. The rest of this section describes coping strategies to help you manage crises as smoothly as possible and avoid symptoms of depression or posttraumatic stress disorder, which are characterized by a more persistent negative mood, flashbacks, and nightmares.

Strategies for Managing OCD Symptoms during a Crisis

Strategy (chapter)	Description
Change your perspective on obsessions (Chapter 3).	Accept that obsessional thoughts will show up, but use strategies like dropping the rope and objectifying the obsession to help you see these thoughts as mental noise, rather than as facts.
Discredit obsessions (Chapter 3).	Use techniques like the life savings wager to step back and recognize that obsessions are based on flawed logic.
Delay your rituals (Chapter 4).	Allow compulsive urges to pass by postponing the ritual or surfing the urge until it subsides.
Modify your rituals (Chapter 4).	Do the ritual incorrectly or incompletely until the urge decreases.
Use distraction and other competing responses (Chapter 4).	Engage in an activity that prevents you from performing the ritual until the urge subsides.
Use positive reinforcement (Chapter 4).	Reward yourself for resisting your compulsive rituals!

Prioritize Balance and Routine

Maintaining a regular routine can provide a sense of normality and control, which may help reduce anxiety about falling behind. Techniques like the ABCD method for minimizing distractions covered in Chapter 5 are particularly useful during stressful times. To effectively manage pressing issues, it might be beneficial to temporarily set aside some daily responsibilities. For example, consider reducing nonessential commitments, and don't shy away from accepting help with tasks like shopping or cooking. It's also okay to take time off from work or school if feasible. This strategy helps conserve energy and reduce stress, facilitating a better handling of both immediate challenges and OCD symptoms.

Remember, during particularly stressful periods, simply making it through the day can be a significant accomplishment. Prioritize essential tasks and responsibilities that are critical for managing the current situation. Allowing yourself to temporarily defer less urgent tasks can relieve pressure and help maintain mental stability. It's crucial to find a balance that respects the need for structure, which provides comfort while adjusting to the demands of the situation. Reflect on and list your priorities, considering ways to simplify or delegate tasks to conserve energy and focus effectively on navigating both the immediate challenges and your mental health needs.

Seek Social Support

As you learned in Chapter 7, assistance from family, friends, or dedicated support groups is not just about getting practical help; it's about having a network of people who understand the complexities posed by the intersection of a crisis and OCD. Family and friends can provide a comforting presence and offer reassurance and understanding to help alleviate your anxiety and stress. They can also help maintain a semblance of normality, assisting when regular routines and tasks become overwhelming. Just knowing that there are people who understand what you're going through and will be patient and supportive can be incredibly grounding. In essence, your support network acts as a crucial buffer against the compounded stress and turmoil of a crisis. It offers emotional comfort, practical assistance, and a sense of shared under-standing and solidarity, all of which are vital to navigating the turbu-lent waters of a crisis compounded by OCD.

Stay Healthy

During a crisis it's particularly important to maintain your diet, sleep, and exercise routines. Sticking to a structured meal plan stabilizes your mood and energy levels and also offers you the comfort of predictabil-ity, easing the stress of food-related decisions. Ensuring consistent sleep patterns is vital too; poor sleep exacerbates stress and OCD symptoms. Creating a calming bedtime routine and a comfortable sleeping envi-ronment helps you get the restorative rest you need to recharge, main-tain emotional resilience, and face challenges with renewed energy and clarity. Engaging in regular physical activity, such as walking or yoga, also acts as a healthy outlet for your anxiety and stress. The endorphins released during exercise naturally boost your mood. These routines act as pillars of stability and control, providing a sense of accomplishment that can be especially valuable when circumstances are overwhelming and chaotic.

Sort Out Your Thoughts and Feelings

Understand that an intensification in your obsessions, compulsions, and anxiety is a normal response during a crisis—not a failure in your man-agement of OCD. One effective way to process your escalated symp-toms is through journaling. Keeping some kind of diary allows you to externalize your thoughts and fears, creating opportunities to reflect on and organize your feelings. Journaling can offer a sense of release and can be a useful tool in tracking patterns or triggers in your OCD symptoms, especially during the heightened stress of a crisis. It serves as a self-awareness exercise, helping you identify and understand the specifics of your increased symptoms and how they relate to the ongo-ing crisis.

Depending on the crisis you're facing, it might also be helpful to talk to a mental health professional. A therapist who understands OCD can help you navigate the intensified symptoms and guide you to a clearer view of your situation. You can also express and process your fears and anxieties related to both the crisis and your OCD without judgment, which not only helps in processing your thoughts, but also contributes to maintaining a level of control over your symptoms during challenging times.

Be Patient and Practice Self-Compassion

As discussed in Chapter 2, embracing self-compassion means being kind to yourself, giving yourself permission to heal at your own pace. Revisit the self-compassion exercises from that chapter, including embracing who you are beyond OCD, focusing on your values and rewarding your resilience. CBT is also an effective tool. Separate from ERP, CBT for stress and crisis management equips you with a structured set of skills for better handling of tumultuous situations. It also offers an approach to recognizing and altering unhelpful thinking patterns that you're susceptible to in the aftermath of a crisis, such as jumping to negative conclusions, engaging in all-or-nothing thinking (as opposed to seeing the nuances), blaming yourself for events you can't control, and focusing excessively on negatives while downplaying your personal strengths.

Part of being patient with yourself involves setting realistic goals and expectations. It's important to celebrate all victories and progress, no matter how minor they may seem. Each step forward, be it successfully managing a trigger or getting through a particularly challenging day, is significant. Remember, recovery is not linear, and there will be ups and downs. The important point is to keep moving forward.

Managing Different Types of Crises

The following section discusses strategies for handling different types of crises—household emergencies and accidents, health-related issues, job loss, and academic problems. The focus is on taking practical steps to gain resilience and clarity so you can navigate the crisis while maintaining control over OCD-related stress.

Household Crises and Accidents

SECURITY CONCERNS

Threats to home security are disturbing for anyone, but if your OCD symptoms include fears of break-ins and compulsive checking of doors, locks, or security-camera footage, then facing real threats like neighborhood burglaries or a robbery at your own home will intensify these anxieties and behaviors. If you find yourself in this situation, it's perfectly reasonable to double-check that all doors and windows are locked securely. For added peace of mind, you might also consider installing a security system. That said, taking these reasonable security measures is generally sufficient to secure your home. So challenge yourself to avoid *excessive* checking as it can feed into OCD fears and behaviors. Repeated checking doesn't increase your safety, but it *does* reinforce your anxiety and sense of danger. Instead, develop a routine for checking doors and windows, perhaps once or twice. If you feel the urge to check again, try delaying the action and distract yourself with another activity for a few minutes. Reward yourself for adhering to your checking limits. By implementing these strategies, you can address security concerns in a way that is effective and mindful of your mental health.

WATER LEAKAGE OR FLOODING

If you have fears of contamination, facing a water leakage or flood can seem like a serious crisis and requires a thoughtful balance between practical action and addressing your OCD symptoms. Initially, pinpoint the source of the leak and, if needed, shut off the main water valve to prevent further water influx. Use towels, mops, or buckets to manage the spread of water effectively. It's crucial to recognize that while cleanliness is important, the situation likely does not warrant excessive cleaning measures. Remind yourself that the presence of water does not necessarily mean the area is contaminated beyond repair. Focus on practical, necessary cleaning and drying methods—perhaps using gloves if wearing them helps mitigate your fears. If the contamination fear is overwhelming, set specific, reasonable limits on cleaning time and intensity, perhaps cleaning the affected area thoroughly once and then allowing it to dry, and resisting the urge to repeatedly clean the same spot. If the urge to keep cleaning persists, use the strategies in Chapter 4 to put off these rituals until the area has dried. In the meantime, try to throw yourself into some other activity as a form of distraction. Remember, the goal is to address the water issue effectively without letting OCD-driven fears dictate your response. If the anxiety becomes unmanageable, consider seeking assistance from a member of your support network such as a family member, friend, or professional who can help ensure that your response remains balanced and practical.

PEST INFESTATION

If you have OCD centered on contamination fears from pests and face a crisis involving a pest infestation in your home, start by acknowledging your anxiety but strive to keep it in perspective. Hire a reputable extermination service to thoroughly treat and document the eradication of the infestation, which will help reassure you of the cleanliness and safety of your environment. Additionally, engage your support network and connect with others who understand your experience and provide insights and encouragement. Such support is vital in helping you navigate the situation without exacerbating your symptoms, offering both practical strategies (perhaps a place to stay while your home is being treated) and emotional reassurance to bolster your ability to cope with the crisis effectively.

CAR ACCIDENTS

Just because you have an excessive fear of accidents doesn't mean they *can't* happen to you! But if your OCD symptoms involve fears of making serious driving mistakes, hitting pedestrians, or causing other mishaps, there are practical strategies you can use to manage your fears in the event such a tragedy actually occurs. First, keep thorough documentation of the incident, including photos and notes, to provide the necessary information to the authorities and to provide you with reassurance. At the same time, try to set limits on your checking behaviors, such as reviewing the accident details only a certain number of times per day and gradually reducing this number. Maintaining your regular routine will help you put the situation into perspective and provide a sense of normality and control, while regular physical activity can help you reduce the stress of such a crisis. Making use of your support system for understanding and coping strategies is important here too. Finally, try to avoid excessive exposure to triggers, such as news stories about car accidents or similar media content, to keep your OCD symptoms from worsening.

Health-Related Crises

RECEIVING A MEDICAL DIAGNOSIS

When dealing with a significant health-related crisis (for yourself or a loved one), it's important to balance staying informed with managing your OCD by using a mix of focused attention and distraction techniques. Begin by educating yourself, but proceed with caution. It's best to gather information directly from your health care providers or from individuals you personally know who have experienced the illness. Be wary of the impulse to search for additional details online—and if you do go online, visit only websites that are known for their credibility and are backed by professional organizations or experts in the field. The information on these sites is regularly updated and fact-checked. If you're going to read posts in public forums or discussion groups (which I don't think is a good idea in the first place), stick with those posts that experts oversee and moderate to ensure that the advice given is reliable and supportive. The danger in seeking out every detail is that your mind will latch on to the worst-case scenarios and most alarming possibilities, even if they are extremely rare, sparking excessive worrying. What's more, unverified or incorrect information can lead to poor decisions regarding your health, safety, or overall well-being.

At the same time, do your best to maintain your daily routine to preserve a sense of control. And, as much as possible, engage in enjoyable activities and social connections to support your emotional well-being. Participating in hobbies and interests that bring you joy can be a vital part of managing the stress of receiving a medical diagnosis. Whether it's reading, painting, hiking, or playing music, these activities provide a valuable distraction and can help divert your mind from constant worries. Keeping in touch with friends and family, whether through face-to-face meetings, video calls, or even messaging, helps reinforce your social network and provides emotional support. Such interactions remind you that you're not alone, offering comfort and perhaps new perspectives on your situation.

SERIOUS INJURY

In the event of an unexpected injury to you or a loved one, your first steps should be to obtain immediate medical care and to diligently follow up with scheduled medical appointments. Coping with this type of crisis can be especially challenging if you have OCD with fears related to accidents and injuries. To manage anxiety during these times, particularly while waiting in medical facilities, incorporate calming practices such as listening to music or podcasts and performing deep breathing exercises. These activities can help mitigate the immediate stress and divert your mind from obsessional thoughts. Also don't hesitate to reach out to your support network—friends, family, or mental health workers—who can provide emotional uplift and practical advice. They're invaluable in helping you navigate the stress of the crisis while keeping your OCD symptoms in check.

If a family member is seriously injured or hospitalized, you'll want to stay informed about their condition and participate in their care. At the same time, schedule regular breaks to safeguard your mental health. Engage in exercises and other activities to help you relax and shift your focus away from the crisis. Such outlets are particularly helpful in managing any heightened anxiety or OCD symptoms related to fears of contamination or hospital environments. Here again, seek out members of your support network to help you maintain a balanced perspective on the situation.

Mistakes and Guilt

If you're grappling with obsessional fears about making financial, legal, medical, or other types of mistakes and you've actually committed such an error, begin with an objective assessment of the situation and any resulting negative outcomes or harm. Discuss the incident with a member of your support network who can offer a balanced perspective.

Remember, even if you've actually slipped up, OCD can amplify feelings of guilt and responsibility, making it important to accurately assess the extent of your accountability and the true scope of the costs.

For example, if you perceive a mistake in your professional work as truly disastrous, your support person can help you scrutinize this belief by comparing it to the facts. This evaluation might include determining the true consequences of the error, considering how others may perceive the situation, and assessing the real probability and seriousness of the worst-case scenarios you imagine. In stepping back and thinking things through, you're likely to find that the situation is not quite as dreadful as it seems. Your support person can then help you reframe your view of the incident. Instead of telling yourself "This mistake is going to ruin my life," they can guide you to a more constructive perspective: "I made a mistake, and I can manage it responsibly and learn from it." This perspective will significantly reduce the emotional burden of the error and help lessen the associated anxiety and guilt. It also promotes resilience by helping you see that errors—even significant ones—do not define your competence or worth, enabling a healthier approach to mishaps when they occur.

When it's clear that you indeed played a significant role in a negative outcome, accept responsibility appropriately. Provide a sincere apology that acknowledges the impact of your mistake and demonstrates genuine remorse. Learn from the experience by analyzing what happened and considering what can be done differently in the future. If your actions have truly caused harm to others, do something to directly address the consequences. Engage in open dialogue by sharing thoughts and feelings and using active listening skills to allow those affected to express their feelings, which can help in rebuilding trust. Provide practical help or compensation if appropriate, such as fixing or replacing damaged items or offering financial reparation. Commit to personal improvement by seeking education or training relevant to the mistake. Follow up to ensure that the resolution is satisfactory and offer emotional support to help alleviate any distress caused. These efforts show your dedication to rectifying the situation and restoring affected relationships. Meanwhile, practice self-compassion and remind yourself of two truths: First, perfection is unattainable—everyone makes mistakes. Second, you are not defined by your mistakes.

Job Loss

To navigate a loss of employment, begin by adopting a structured plan that addresses both your immediate needs and your OCD-related fears about the future. Start by updating your résumé and any online profiles, such as LinkedIn. Then dedicate time for job searching and networking to help you maintain a sense of routine and purpose. Set achievable goals, such as applying to a specific number of jobs each week, and work on developing new skills that are relevant to your field. Enrolling in online courses or workshops can enhance your skill set and boost your confidence. To manage OCD-related anxieties, maintain a progress journal to track your development and visually affirm your capabilities.

It never hurts to expand your professional network by reaching out to former coworkers, joining professional groups, or attending networking events. Use positive affirmations to overcome any social anxiety or fears about reaching out. Finally, maintain a balanced diet, adequate sleep, and regular exercise to support your overall well-being during this period. These strategies will help you tackle practical aspects of finding new employment and also support your mental health, keeping you grounded and prepared for new opportunities.

Academic Crises

Navigating serious academic problems, such as failing a class or facing the prospect of failing out of school, can be especially stressful when you're dealing with OCD. To manage such a crisis, start by setting up a meeting with your academic advisor or professors to discuss your current situation and explore possible solutions, such as retaking courses or adjusting your course load. Acknowledge your concerns about your academic performance but counter them with practical steps to improve. For example, develop a realistic study plan that includes scheduled study times, breaks, and specific goals for each session. This structure can help provide you with a sense of control.

Especially if your OCD and anxiety symptoms focus on perfectionism or the fear of failure, remember that a single academic setback does not define your entire academic career, let alone your future.

School can be a challenging environment, and it's not uncommon for many students, whether they have OCD or not, to face difficulties at some point in their educational journey. You likely know of people who have faced academic challenges yet ultimately achieved success over time—this is quite common. Their stories highlight the fact that long-term success is often shaped not just by academic performance but by resilience, adaptability, and continuous effort.

Look at it this way: Experiencing academic challenges can provide valuable lessons in perseverance, problem solving, and self-advocacy. It teaches you how to bounce back from disappointments and better prepares you for future obstacles. By addressing and overcoming these difficulties, you gain a deeper understanding of your own strengths and weaknesses, which is important for personal and professional growth. Thus, while it may feel disheartening at the moment, navigating these challenges can set the foundation for a resilient and successful path forward. Remember, your response to adversity can be a powerful determinant of your future success.

In the meantime, work to enhance your learning strategies by attending academic workshops, utilizing school resources like tutoring centers, and forming study groups. These resources can offer new approaches to learning and support from peers who might be facing similar challenges. Also, be sure to maintain a balanced lifestyle with adequate sleep, nutrition, and exercise, as physical well-being significantly impacts mental and cognitive performance.

Finally, if you feel that OCD symptoms are significantly impacting your ability to study effectively, consider seeking support from a counselor or mental health professional with experience in helping people manage academic pressures. If you haven't already, this is also a good time to explore the possibility of academic accommodations, as discussed in Chapter 10. By taking proactive steps and tapping available resources, you can address the root causes of your academic difficulties and set a path toward recovery and success in your educational endeavors. Keep in mind that reaching out for help and advocating for your needs is a sign of strength, not weakness, and it can make a crucial difference in managing both your educational and mental health challenges.

Facing a crisis causes significant disruption and heightens stress and anxiety—both of which are compounded by OCD. But by using the strategies you've learned to manage obsessions and compulsions, by prioritizing essential tasks, by engaging in calming activities, and by leveraging your support network, you can maintain control and balance, and successfully navigate these challenges. Your support network is especially important because it not only offers practical assistance, but also emotional comfort, which is critical during stressful periods. By maintaining your routine, you reinforce your resilience and enhance your capacity to handle adversity. While getting through a crisis is indeed challenging, it's also an opportunity for personal growth. The skills and insights you develop in these difficult times will not only help you manage the current situation but also improve your capacity to tackle future challenges, ultimately cultivating a more resilient and stronger self.

Practical Steps for Living Well: Surviving a Crisis

Plan for crises:

- Understand how crises can exacerbate OCD symptoms.
- Prepare crisis management strategies in advance.

Maintain your routine:

- Stick to a regular schedule to preserve your sense of normality and control.
- Prioritize essential tasks and responsibilities over nonessential ones.
- Practice self-care and prioritize healthy diet, sleep, and exercise routines.

Sort out your thoughts and feelings:

- Keep a journal to process your thoughts and fears during a crisis.
- Get perspective and support for your feelings from someone you trust.

Practice self-compassion:

- Recognize that increased OCD symptoms during a crisis are normal.
- Celebrate small victories and progress and remember that recovery is not linear.

12

rethinking treatment

In Chapter 1, you learned that exposure and response prevention (ERP) is the gold standard treatment for OCD. Over 50 years of research has demonstrated its ability to weaken the vicious cycle of obsessions and compulsions by helping you do two things that OCD usually discourages you from doing:[1] (1) confront your fears (the exposure component) and (2) abstain from your usual ritualistic behaviors (the response prevention component). The core therapy involves working with a trained mental health professional who teams up with you to develop a treatment plan and then coaches you through the ERP practice. The treatment aims to show you that you don't need to perform compulsive rituals or avoid fear-provoking situations to cope with obsessional anxiety, effectively diminishing OCD's influence over your life.

But ERP is challenging work, and, understandably, most people with OCD aren't exactly thrilled about facing their fears and giving up their rituals. Many ultimately decide that doing so is worthwhile since

---

[1] Although ERP has been applied to OCD for 50 years, the principles underlying exposure therapy have been studied and used to treat people with all sorts of fears and phobias for over a century.

the chances are good that in the long run it will result in fewer OCD symptoms and a better quality of life. However, some people refuse this treatment. And even though it works for most people, some who try it don't achieve the response they were hoping for.

This chapter aims to help you resolve both issues: (1) overcoming your reluctance to start or continue ERP and (2) enhancing the effectiveness of ERP if you're already undergoing treatment. If you haven't tried ERP or stopped it prematurely, you'll discover strategies to overcome your hesitation and see how this treatment can reduce symptoms and improve your quality of life. If you feel you're not benefiting enough from ERP, the later section "Strategies for Long-Term Success" offers techniques to maximize the treatment's long-term effectiveness. In some instances, the same strategies will be beneficial for both challenges. Overall, this chapter provides insights and tools to help you navigate the treatment process with confidence and resilience. It will debunk myths that may prevent engagement with ERP, clarify what the therapy entails, and address common obstacles.

ERP Myths and Misunderstandings

Given the challenging nature of ERP, misconceptions about this therapy are understandable. So let's begin by debunking the most common myths. As you read this section, consider whether these misconceptions have kept you from trying ERP. If you're currently in therapy, or have tried it previously, reflect on whether they've interfered with your success. By gaining a clear understanding of what ERP actually involves, you can form realistic expectations and better navigate the natural highs and lows of the process without becoming discouraged.

Myth 1: ERP Is Too Harsh or Extreme to Be Helpful

The idea that ERP is excessive, cruel, dangerous, or will make your OCD worse overlooks the controlled and rational nature of this therapy. While it's true that you'll almost certainly feel distress if you're doing ERP properly, this distress is temporary. What's more, the temporary distress is an important aspect of the treatment that leads to long-term benefits. It's also important to know that no one is ever forced to do exposure therapy—that would be completely unethical! Your therapist will *suggest* or *challenge* you to face your fears, but the decision to do so is entirely yours in the end. ERP is also not about provoking as much pain or distress as possible and then making you sit with it. It's about helping you face your fears with compassionate coaching, allowing you to gradually build resilience and reduce your anxiety over time.

How exactly does exposure therapy work? For one thing, as you consistently confront your fears and resist relying on compulsive rituals, you gradually become less sensitive to your fear triggers—a well-studied psychological process known as *habituation*. Essentially, ERP reduces the association between your triggers and your anxiety. If you have successfully tackled other everyday fears in the past by facing them head on, you're familiar with how this mechanism works. Additionally, facing your fears boosts your sense of empowerment by demonstrating that anxiety is safe, temporary, and manageable, which in turn builds your resilience and confidence. As you practice more and more, the grip of OCD loosens and you find yourself better able to engage fully in life. You may stop avoiding situations that triggered OCD symptoms in the past or open up time in your day for what you want to do by cutting down on checking rituals. Extensive research supports ERP's effectiveness, highlighting that despite initial discomfort, the lasting benefits of this approach significantly contribute to long-term mental health and functioning.

Myth 2: ERP Doesn't Address the Underlying Issues at Work

ERP does not explore issues related to your childhood or your subconscious. While these deep-seated psychological factors may influence OCD on some level, research shows that addressing them is not required to reduce obsessions and compulsions. Instead, ERP addresses three important "here-and-now" factors that decades of research clearly link to OCD:

- The tendency to think that your obsessional fears are likely to come true
- The tendency to respond to obsessional fear as if you are truly in danger
- The tendency to view uncertainty and anxiety (along with other feelings such as disgust) as unmanageable or unsafe

Myth 3: ERP Is Just Like Facing Your Fears on Your Own

My patients sometimes mention that they engage in ERP "all the time" without seeing results. Further discussion, however, usually reveals that their experiences were not genuine ERP but rather unplanned and unwelcome encounters with fear-triggering situations. During these encounters, they performed compulsions or used subtle (or not so subtle) avoidance tactics to try to minimize anxious feelings. But this differs from the way a therapist would guide ERP sessions. Actual therapeutic ERP involves repeated *planned, intentional* confrontations with your fears in a controlled and supportive setting. It also requires a trained therapist to guide you and promote the therapeutic changes needed to reduce your OCD symptoms.

Myth 4: I'll Have to "Sit with My Anxiety" during Exposure

The idea that you'll have to face your fears and then just "sit there," passively waiting for your anxiety to go away, is a common misconception. In reality, your therapist will encourage you to engage actively in your daily activities *alongside* your anxiety, rather than avoiding them because of anxious feelings or waiting around for them to go away. This proactive approach helps you learn that anxiety and obsessions don't need to dictate your actions or stop you from doing what matters most in your life. Your therapist will help you develop new, constructive responses to anxiety that do not rely on compulsive behaviors. The aim is to empower you with the confidence and skills to lead a fulfilling life, even when intrusive thoughts, uncertainty, and anxiety are present.

Myth 5: Improvement Should Be Immediate

Would you sit behind the wheel of a car for the first time and expect to expertly navigate busy city traffic? Would you pick up a guitar and expect to be able to strum your favorite tune perfectly on the first try? It's the same with overcoming problems like OCD. Just like learning how to drive and play a musical instrument, true progress with ERP is seen over a period of consistent practice. So don't expect it to occur immediately. ERP is the kind of active and skills-based treatment where the more time and effort you invest, the greater the rewards.

Myth 6: ERP Is Effective Only for Mild OCD

Extensive research shows that ERP can significantly reduce OCD symptoms across all levels of severity, including moderate to severe cases. The treatment process can be challenging and may initially increase anxiety, but it ultimately weakens the link between obsessive thoughts and compulsive actions. For severe symptoms, a comprehensive treatment plan that may include more intense therapy sessions (perhaps in a residential program), longer treatment duration, and integration with other treatments like medication that is often effective.

Myth 7: Success in ERP Means Completely Eliminating Anxiety

By now it should be clear that the main objective of ERP isn't to completely eliminate anxiety but rather to help you manage it more effectively. Anxiety is a natural part of human experience, and expecting it to vanish entirely is both unrealistic and unproductive. ERP focuses on diminishing the *power* of anxiety and obsessional thoughts by demonstrating that you can still function effectively despite them. When you gain this confidence, anxiety naturally decreases—although it won't go away entirely. *As I like to say, the goal of ERP is to help you get better at **having** anxiety, not get better at making it go away.*

But ERP Still Seems Too Daunting!

Imagine you're at the base of a mountain, looking up at the peak. You know reaching the top will offer breathtaking views and a sense of accomplishment, but the steep, rocky path ahead makes you hesitate. Starting ERP can feel similar. The climb looks daunting. You're apprehensive about the challenge. However, just as each step up the mountain gets you closer to the summit, each exposure practice moves you closer to mastering your fears and loosening OCD's grip on your life. The climb may be tough, but the view from the top is worth it. If you've seriously considered ERP but found yourself unable to actually get started, you're not alone. Many people feel overwhelmed by the idea of directly facing their fears and hesitate to take the first step. In this section, we'll look at common reasons for this hesitation and explore steps you can take to help you overcome them and begin moving forward.

Common Roadblocks to Engaging in ERP

Even if you don't avoid ERP because of subscribing to the preceding myths, you may have other reasons for reluctance. Which of the following reasons resonate with your experiences?

THE FEAR FACTOR

The number-one reason people avoid ERP is that it requires you to confront your fears without the compulsive rituals you typically rely on to control anxiety. Avoiding pain and discomfort is an innate instinct and perfectly understandable. In the case of OCD, however, automatically obeying this instinct keeps you trapped in a lower quality of life than you deserve. Do fears that your obsessions will become reality hold you back? Are you worried the anxiety will be unbearable or spiral out of control? In truth, the most intense discomfort is typically short lived. What's more, you possess more strength and resilience than you realize, and you are likely to find yourself handling these challenges more capably than you expected. The section on strategies for overcoming roadblocks gives you a chance to prove this to yourself.

UNDERESTIMATING OCD

Acknowledging the severity of your OCD can be difficult. You might play down its impact on your life or believe that you can control it without professional help. This thinking can be a significant barrier to engaging in ERP. After all, why undergo a challenging therapy if you believe OCD is manageable your own?

LIMITED AWARENESS OF OCD SYMPTOMS

A related roadblock is what mental health professionals call *poor insight,* which means not fully recognizing that your obsessions and compulsions are out of proportion to the actual risks or dangers they are meant to guard against. If you believe your obsessional fears are rational or your rituals are necessary to prevent disaster, doing ERP will seem unsafe or irresponsible.

ACCOMMODATIONS BY WELL-MEANING OTHERS

Accommodation of your OCD by family or friends can reduce your incentive to pursue change, especially through a challenging therapy like ERP. For instance, if your sibling always drives the car to avoid the fear of hitting pedestrians, you might not feel the need to confront this fear through exposures. If your partner provides constant reassurance, you may be less inclined to work on stopping your reassurance-seeking rituals. And if your family helps cover expenses, allowing you not to work, you might not see the necessity of doing ERP to manage your symptoms and seek employment. But of course, you also don't get to enjoy the independence of driving yourself, the confidence of managing your own anxiety, or the fulfillment of being self-sufficient. The comfort and ease that such accommodations offer can diminish your motivation to do the challenging work of ERP—while also diminishing your life.

FEAR OF CHANGE

Believe it or not, *recovery* from OCD can also be a source of anxiety. As you improve, you may have new expectations of yourself, and expectations from others may arise. You might worry about handling increased responsibilities at work or school or in personal relationships once you're no longer viewed as someone struggling with OCD. The familiarity of the status quo might feel more comfortable than stepping into the uncertainties of a new lifestyle, making the idea of change seem daunting.

HOPELESSNESS AND DEPRESSION

If you've been battling OCD for a long time, you may believe that improvement is unattainable. Past unsuccessful treatment efforts might have also fostered a sense of pessimism regarding your chances of recovery. These feelings can make the effort required to do ERP seem pointless. Additionally, if you are dealing with depression, you might feel undeserving of improvement. Together these factors create a substantial obstacle to initiating treatment.

PAST NEGATIVE EXPERIENCES WITH ERP

Have you had a bad experience trying ERP in the past? If your therapist wasn't properly trained or ERP was executed ineffectively, it could lead to distrust in the treatment process, making it difficult to commit to trying ERP again. If you were not given sufficient support in the past, the fear of repeating such experiences may discourage you from pursuing the therapy again. If you were pushed into trying ERP by a parent or significant other before you were ready, you might have negative associations with this treatment. Any of these factors can lead to reluctance to engage in ERP, despite its potential benefits.

Strategies for Overcoming Roadblocks and Embracing ERP

If any of these obstacles seem familiar, know that they don't have to continue to stand in the way of your living well. Here are some strategies to implement, beginning with the easiest and most straightforward, that can help you address the challenges and reconsider engaging in ERP or engage in it more thoroughly.

EDUCATION

Dispelling the myths covered earlier in this chapter and familiarizing yourself with the substantial scientific evidence supporting ERP's effectiveness can bolster your confidence in this approach. You can use free internet search engines like Google Scholar to get access to research studies or to read summaries of the literature on websites such as the IOCDF (*www.iocdf.org*). By deepening your knowledge of ERP, you're better equipped to approach it with a positive and informed perspective, ready to tackle its challenges head-on.

TAKE A GRADUAL APPROACH

If it's fear of exposure that's made you hesitant, taking it a little more slowly might be helpful. Develop an even more gradual hierarchy or "ladder" of exposure situations than what ERP typically suggests (or than what you've tried before if you've dabbled in ERP)—on your own or with your therapist—and begin with those exposures that still challenge your OCD but do not feel overwhelming. As you gain confidence, gradually increase the difficulty. You don't need to be in a hurry to get there because taking your time allows you to build a solid foundation of coping skills, ensuring that each step is firmly established before moving on to more challenging tasks. This steady progression not only enhances your resilience, but also minimizes the risk of overwhelming yourself, making the process more manageable and effective.

ADDRESS PAST NEGATIVE EXPERIENCES

If you've previously had unfavorable experiences with ERP, make it a priority to discuss them openly with your therapist. Such conversations can reveal insights into what may have gone wrong, such as a mismatch with the therapist, too rapid a pace of exposure, and inadequate support. By analyzing these factors, you and your therapist can make the necessary adjustments to avoid past pitfalls. Working together to tailor treatment this way can boost your confidence and transform your perception of ERP from a source of apprehension to a well-organized path toward recovery.

INVOLVE YOUR SUPPORT NETWORK

In Chapter 7 you learned about the importance of educating your family and friends about OCD. Helping them understand what ERP is and how it works enables them to become knowledgeable supporters who understand the dos and don'ts that aid in recovery. The Understanding Exposure and Response Prevention (ERP) for OCD handout on pages 189–190 is a resource you can share with family and friends to teach them about ERP and their role in your recovery. Review it together to address any questions and to assure yourself that they can provide informed, effective support. If your family would benefit from even more detailed information, I've also written an entire book, *The Family Guide to Getting Over OCD,* that provides comprehensive education and strategies for supporting someone with OCD. OCD support groups (as described in Chapter 7) may also be especially helpful since they provide a community of people who share similar experiences, offer emotional support, and suggest practical tips and strategies for getting the most out of ERP. Being part of an informed support system reduces feelings of isolation and creates a safe and encouraging environment through similar success stories, bolstering your confidence to engage with ERP and helping you persist through challenging moments in therapy.

FIND THE RIGHT THERAPIST

To help you confidently embrace ERP, you need a therapist who is both adept at implementing this treatment and has a communication style that aligns with your preferences. A well-trained and highly skilled clinician understands the unique challenges that OCD presents and can customize ERP to fit your individual needs, including adjusting the pace of treatment so that you're ready for each step. If you're

UNDERSTANDING EXPOSURE AND RESPONSE PREVENTION FOR OCD

Exposure and response prevention (ERP) is a type of cognitive-behavioral therapy designed to treat OCD. Individuals face feared situations while resisting the usual compulsive responses. With practice, this exposure reduces anxiety and improves coping skills.

How Does ERP Work?

1. **Assessment and planning:** The therapist and person with OCD identify the obsessions and compulsions. Together they list feared situations, from least to most anxiety provoking.

2. **Exposure:** The therapist coaches the person with OCD through gradually facing their fears in a controlled environment, usually starting with the least-distressing situations.

3. **Response prevention:** The therapist helps the person with OCD resist compulsive behaviors.

4. **Habituation:** Over time, being exposed to feared situations without engaging in compulsions disrupts the cycle of obsession and compulsion and decreases anxiety and distress.

Key Points about ERP

- ERP is carefully structured and supervised, with the therapist providing support throughout.

- Temporary distress leads to significant long-term benefits.

- The therapist encourages and challenges the person with OCD, but never forces them to engage in exposures.

- The goal is to experience manageable levels of anxiety that gradually decrease over time.

(continued)

How Can You Support Your Loved One?

Educate yourself: Learn about OCD and ERP so you understand your loved one's experience.

Support treatment: Encourage your loved one to stick with ERP even when it gets tough.

Avoid accommodation: Avoid assisting with rituals and avoidance, which reinforce OCD.

Provide emotional support: Offer empathy and patience. Acknowledge the smallest efforts.

Respect boundaries: Understand that ERP is a personal journey. Respect your loved one's pace and boundaries.

What Are the Benefits of ERP?

Reduces anxiety and distress: Over time, ERP helps reduce the anxiety and distress associated with OCD.

Improves quality of life: By understanding and supporting ERP, you can play a role in your loved one's journey toward managing OCD. Successful ERP can lead to a more fulfilling and less restricted life.

shopping around for a new therapist, don't hesitate to ask about a therapist's professional credentials and experience right up front—mental health practitioners are accustomed to these questions. Similarly, if you're concerned that your current therapist may lack the necessary skills, it's perfectly fine to respectfully bring up this concern and consider a referral to someone with more expertise. For example, you might say, "I've been thinking about my progress, and I wonder if I might benefit from seeing someone with more specialized experience in OCD and ERP. Could we discuss the possibility of a referral?" It's important that you feel confident in your therapist's ability to effectively guide you through the therapy process and that you also feel a sense of trust and openness with your therapist. You should feel comfortable relying on them for empathy, support, and encouragement, which are essential for sustaining your commitment and helping you face your fears.

FIND THE RIGHT SETTING

Finding a therapeutic setting that matches your comfort level with ERP can make the treatment less daunting and unlock your ability to engage. Options like self-help resources or outpatient therapy are ideal if you prefer a flexible and less intensive starting point. Group therapy adds the benefit of peer support and motivation through shared experiences. If your OCD symptoms are more severe, intensive outpatient programs or residential treatment can provide a higher level of structured support, frequent professional care, and complementary therapies alongside ERP, creating a highly supervised and supportive therapeutic environment.

DEFUSE DEPRESSION

Although depression can drain your energy and diminish your motivation for ERP, it can be managed alongside or prior to your OCD treatment. Therapists may use a mix of strategies such as cognitive therapy and a schedule of pleasant activities (sometimes called *behavioral activation therapy*) to enhance your mood. Improving your mood can boost your energy and positivity, making it easier to tackle ERP's anxiety-inducing tasks. Treatment for depression might also include antidepressants, which can alleviate OCD symptoms as well. By treating both conditions together, you can achieve better overall results. It's important to maintain open communication with your therapist about how depression affects your ERP therapy, ensuring that your treatment plan is tailored to your specific needs for more effective support.

FOCUS ON THE LONG TERM AND KEEP MOVING FORWARD

Doing ERP is a lot like moving through a swamp. In the moment, you might feel stuck in the mud, focusing on the anxiety and discomfort that come with facing your fears. It's unpleasant and challenging, just like wading through a thick, murky swamp. However, you're in the swamp for a reason: There's something valuable to be gained on the other side—a greater control over OCD symptoms and a more fulfilling life—that you can reach only by moving through it.

This swamp, with all its discomfort, represents the short-term distress of ERP; but it's crucial for your long-term recovery. Each step forward, though it might increase your anxiety momentarily, is a step toward solid ground. By keeping your focus on the valuable outcomes waiting for you, you can find the incentive to persist through the swamp. It's not just about enduring discomfort but moving toward something that matters deeply to you. Embracing this perspective can transform how you view the immediate challenges of ERP, highlighting them as necessary and worthwhile parts of the journey to recovery.

What If ERP Isn't Working?

The success of ERP can differ depending on how the therapy is implemented and practiced. Therefore, getting disappointing results doesn't necessarily mean the treatment is ineffective. It might simply suggest that some adjustments are needed. Here are several strategies for optimizing your approach.

Practice Consistently, but Don't Overdo It

As previously mentioned, progressing in ERP is like developing any new skill—it requires consistent practice. Your therapist (or self-help guide) will provide instructions for how to thoughtfully conduct your exposure practices, including how frequently to repeat them. Adhering to this program and being methodical about doing exposure practices are important for success. Skipping steps or reverting to old habits can reinforce OCD symptoms and hinder your progress.

In a similar vein, don't go overboard with ERP! Exposure therapy is a powerful tool, but only when it's used properly. I've seen people who initially see benefits with exposure but then use it as a tool for quickly alleviating their anxiety whenever they experience an obsession. This habit is detrimental because it transforms the treatment into a compulsive ritual. Remember that the primary goal of ERP is to help you learn to *manage* obsessional fear and anxiety, not to *eliminate* them. So never use exposure just to make your anxiety go away. Doing so will disrupt the learning process and keep you stuck in OCD's vicious cycle. If you think you might be overusing exposure, it's important to discuss this tendency with your therapist to ensure that you're following the treatment correctly and effectively.

Use Mindfulness and Acceptance

When we label experiences like anxiety and obsessional thoughts as "bad" or "unwanted," we create resistance that only amplifies the distress. So instead, try changing how you *relate* to these thoughts and feelings by incorporating mindfulness and acceptance into your ERP treatment. Mindfulness encourages observing thoughts and feelings without attaching judgments or reacting impulsively, allowing you to acknowledge your experiences without escalating them. For instance, while you're confronting a fear-provoking situation, try incorporating strategies from Chapter 3, such as dropping the rope, to help you observe your reactions with openness and nonjudgment instead of try-ing to change or challenge them. Chapter 4 also includes strategies derived from mindfulness approaches, such as surfing the urge to ritu-alize. It is this welcoming approach to obsessional thoughts, anxiety, and compulsive urges that, over time, helps bring about a more long-lasting reduction in OCD symptoms and improvements in your quality of life.

Embrace the Challenge

ERP can seem intimidating and counterintuitive, especially if you're already feeling hesitant or afraid. Embracing the process can be more manageable with the right mind-set and strategies. Start by focusing on the long-term benefits, rather than on the short-term distress: Con-fronting your fears through ERP helps reinforce mental resilience, fos-tering a more adaptive response to stressors and reducing the overall impact of OCD on your life. Set small goals by breaking down the process into manageable steps to gradually build your confidence. Cel-ebrate small victories along the way to stay engaged. By approaching ERP with these strategies, you can make the commitment less over-whelming and more achievable, paving the way for stronger, long-lasting mental health.

Engage with Your Support System

You can boost the effectiveness of your ERP by involving your support network. Discuss with your therapist the possibility of including a fam-ily member or close friend in your therapy sessions. This both enhances emotional support and educates your loved ones about your experi-ences, increasing their ability to support you. Even if they cannot be present in the therapy sessions, review the handout on pages 189–190, keep your family member or friend informed about your progress, and guide them on specific ways they can assist you. They may be able to accompany you during exposure tasks, help you resist compulsive behaviors, or refrain from offering reassurance. Additionally, maintain-ing regular check-ins with your support network can bolster your com-mitment to therapy and help you remain engaged and proactive.

Anticipate Setbacks

Setbacks and other obstacles are a normal part of the ERP process. So, if you find yourself too anxious to complete an exposure or unable to resist performing rituals, don't panic. Instead of viewing any setback as a failure, look at it as an opportunity to learn and modify your strategy. Openly discuss any setbacks with your therapist, who can assist in fine-tuning your techniques and making necessary adjustments. Remember, each challenge you overcome is a step forward in gaining better control over your OCD and taking back your life.

Strategies for Long-Term Success

ERP is a short-term therapy, typically lasting a few months. But it's designed to equip you with lifelong skills for managing fear and compulsive urges. The aim is to prepare you to be your own therapist, maintaining and building on the improvements made during therapy. If you've successfully finished a course of ERP, the strategies in this section will help you sustain and enhance your improvement.

Ongoing Self-Directed ERP

After the structured therapy ends, it's important to continue practicing ERP exercises on your own. Working with your therapist to develop a personalized routine that includes daily or weekly tasks to confront OCD triggers can help you maintain control over symptoms. These self-directed exercises ensure that you remain proactive about OCD, reducing the likelihood of relapse.

Check In with Yourself Regularly

Set up regular check-ins with yourself—like once a week at the same time—to assess your OCD symptoms. These check-ins can serve as a personal audit on your mental health, helping ensure that you catch any potential setbacks early and address them before they develop further.

Keeping a journal or log, like the Ritual Awareness Log described in Chapter 4, can be a useful way to track your thoughts, feelings, and compulsive behaviors. Seeing your progress written down serves as an excellent motivating factor for continuing to apply ERP and for remembering to contact your therapist if you hit an especially rough patch.

Stay Connected to Professionals

Long-term management of you OCD may involve a combination of continued therapy and possibly medication management. Regularly scheduled therapy sessions, even if less frequent, can help reinforce the use of ERP techniques and provide ongoing support. Additionally, staying educated about OCD and its treatments, participating in support groups, and possibly engaging in maintenance sessions with a therapist can provide ongoing reinforcement and help manage symptoms effectively.

Recognize Lapses and Prevent Relapses

Even when treatment is successful, you'll want to stay alert for lapses—temporary setbacks that might include the return of old behaviors, increased anxiety, or feeling overwhelmed by symptoms that were previously under control. But remember that lapses are normal and not a cause for panic; they simply mean you need to do some exposures and implement response prevention to get things back under control. Ignoring lapses, on the other hand, could lead to *relapse*—a more profound return of obsessions, compulsions, and interference with functioning.

As you move forward from this chapter, embrace the journey of ERP as a dynamic and ongoing process. Remember that mastering these skills is not about achieving perfection but about persistence, education, and adaptability. Recognize that lapses are a normal part of this journey and view them as opportunities to reinforce your ERP strategies rather than as setbacks. By staying vigilant, regularly practicing the techniques you've learned, and maintaining an open line of communication with your therapist and support network, you can continue to manage OCD effectively. Keep educating yourself, involve your loved ones, and stay committed to the long-term maintenance of your mental health. Your journey with ERP is about building resilience and fostering a fulfilling life despite the presence of anxiety and obsessions.

Practical Steps for Living Well: Rethinking Treatment

Educate yourself:

- Get to know how ERP works by using resources like the IOCDF website.
- Discard myths and misinformation to build confidence in the treatment.

Incorporate strategies to optimize success:

- Work on a ladder of exposure situations with your therapist and practice consistently.
- Make sure family and friends know what you're trying to do so they can support your treatment.
- Talk to others with similar experiences for support and practical tips.

Address challenges head-on:

- Be candid with your therapist to resolve any difficulties with ERP.
- Use mindfulness to observe your thoughts and feelings without judgment.

Prepare for the long term:

- Create a personalized routine for self-directed ERP exercises to prevent relapse.
- Use regular self-assessments to track progress and address any setbacks early.

index

Note. *f* following a page number indicates a figure.

ABCD method strategy, 72–74, 167
Academic functioning. *See* School
    functioning
Acceptance, 193–194. *See also* Self-acceptance
Acceptance and commitment therapy (ACT),
    26–27, 36
Accidents, 171–172, 173. *See also* Crisis
    management
Accommodations
    common work and school
      accommodations, 154, 155
    exposure and response prevention and, 185
    legal rights to in school or work settings,
      154–160
    OCD-related family conflicts and, 125,
      129
    overview, 5
    requesting from employers, 156–158,
      159–160, 163
    requesting from schools, 158, 159–160,
      163, 176
    romantic relationships and, 132, 140–145,
      148
Accountability, 64–65
Active listening, 119–122, 126, 129, 146,
    148. *See also* Communication
Activities. *See also* Enjoyable activities;
    Schedules; Time management
    ABCD method strategy and, 72–74
    as a distraction from compulsive urges,
      60–61

family relationships and, 129
    overcoming procrastination and, 79–81
    recovering from a breakup and, 147
    romantic relationships and, 141, 143, 148
    selecting rewards from, 64
    social activities, 106–107
    structuring days and, 74–77, 82
Activity Log, 69–72, 82
Acts of service, 33, 35
Advocacy groups, 103, 104–105, 161. *See also*
    Support networks
Affirmations, 25–26, 29
Alarms, 73
Americans with Disabilities Act (ADA), 88,
    155
Anti-rituals strategy, 59–60
Anxiety. *See also* Obsessions
    academic crises and, 175–176
    crises and, 5, 177
    cycle of isolation and, 105
    explaining to others, 90–91, 92
    exposure and response prevention and, 18,
      181–183
    overview, 1, 8, 9
    procrastination and, 79
    romantic relationships and, 132, 144
    self-compassion and self-acceptance and,
      23
Arguments, 124–128. *See also* Conflicts
Arranging rituals, 10, 59. *See also*
    Compulsions and compulsive rituals

Avoidance. *See also* Compulsions and
    compulsive rituals; Symptoms
  Activity Log and, 71
  cycle of OCD and, 11–15, 15*f*
  exposure and response prevention and, 17,
    18, 182
  negative reinforcement loop and, 13–14,
    15*f*
  OCD within the family context and, 116
  overview, 2–3, 8–11
  reducing OCD symptoms and, 16
  romantic relationships and, 142

Behavioral activation therapy, 191–192
Behaviors. *See* Compulsions and compulsive
    rituals; Rituals
Boundaries
  building a support network and, 100, 101
  dealing with negativity and, 110, 111–112,
    114
  romantic relationships and, 136, 148
  sharing your OCD story and, 86, 91–93,
    95–96
  time management and, 78
Brainstorming solutions, 123. *See also*
    Decision making; Problem solving
Breaking down tasks, 75, 80–81, 151–152,
    163. *See also* Prioritizing tasks; Time
    management
Breaks, taking, 75–76, 153, 173
Breakups, 146–147. *See also* Romantic
    relationships
Breathing exercises, 153, 173

Calendar use, 74–77, 152–153. *See also*
    Schedules; Time management
Car accidents, 171–172. *See also* Crisis
    management
Celebrating progress, 63–65, 80, 144,
    161–162, 178
Checking behaviors, 10, 59, 170. *See also*
    Compulsions and compulsive rituals
Clarification, 120–121, 122–123
Cleaning, 10, 131–132. *See also* Compulsions
    and compulsive rituals
Cognitive-behavioral therapy (CBT), 1, 16,
    169. *See also* Treatment
Communication. *See also* Sharing your OCD
    story with others
  active listening, 119–122, 129, 146, 148
  boundaries and, 111–112
  building a support network and, 101–103
  cycle of isolation and, 106

  dealing with negativity and, 111–112
  family communication patterns, 118–124,
    128, 129
  habits to avoid in, 121–122
  "I" statements, 90, 112–113, 118–119, 127,
    129
  OCD-related family conflicts and,
    124–128
  overview, 5, 11
  problem solving and decision making and,
    122–124
  responding to reactions from others,
    93–96
  romantic relationships and, 133, 136, 139,
    146, 148
  sharing your OCD story and, 90–93, 98
Community, 86, 96–97, 103–104, 109–110.
    See also Support networks
Compassion. *See* Self-compassion
Competing responses, 58–61, 166
Compromise, 127, 129
Compulsions and compulsive rituals. *See also*
    Avoidance; Mental rituals; Patterns;
    Rituals; Symptoms
  Activity Log and, 71
  awareness of, 52–55, 53*f*
  competing responses and, 58–61, 66
  crises and, 165, 169–176
  cycle of OCD and, 11–15, 15*f*
  delaying, 55–57, 66
  explaining to others, 90–91, 92
  exposure and response prevention and,
    16–18, 182
  modifying, 57–58, 66
  negative reinforcement loop and, 13–14
  overview, 4, 8–11, 51, 65, 66
  positive reinforcement and, 63–65
  rewarding yourself for, 66
  romantic relationships and, 131–132,
    137–139, 148
  support from others and, 61–63, 66
Confession rituals, 136, 139
Confidence, 63, 138–139
Confidentiality, 159
Conflicts, 5, 116–117, 124–128, 145–147
Connection, 87–88. *See also* Relationships;
    Support networks
Contamination fears, 9, 131, 137, 170–171
Coping strategies. *See also individual strategies*
  crises and, 165–169
  negative reinforcement loop and, 13–14
  OCD within the family context and, 116
  reducing accommodations within a
    romantic relationship and, 144
  rewarding resilience and, 31

Core values
    overview, 26–29, 27f, 34, 35
    prioritizing tasks and, 68
    procrastination and, 79
Crisis management
    academic crises, 175–176
    effects of OCD on, 165
    health-related crises, 172–173
    household crises and accidents, 170–172
    job loss, 175
    mistakes and guilt, 173–174
    overview, 5, 164, 177, 178
    strategies for managing OCD with,
        165–169
    types of crises and, 169–176
Criticism from others, 110–113, 121–122
Cycle of OCD, 11–15, 15f, 62–63

Dating, 5, 11, 87–88. See also Romantic
    relationships
Decision making
    family communication patterns and,
        122–124
    OCD-related family conflicts and,
        126–128
    romantic relationships and, 146
    understanding of OCD and, 7
Delaying rituals, 55–57, 137, 166
Depression, 1, 18, 186, 191–192
Diet, 168, 178
Digital tools, 74–77, 89, 152–153
Disagreements. See Arguments; Conflicts
Disapproval from others, 95–96, 110–113
Disclosure. See Sharing your OCD story
    with others
Discrediting obsessions
    crises and, 166
    overview, 42–49, 50
    reasoning behind obsessions, 43–45
    relationship OCD (ROCD) and, 138–139
    transforming the narrative and, 45–49
Distraction strategy, 60–61, 166
Distractions, minimizing, 77–78, 82
Distress, emotional. See Emotional distress
Doubts, 8, 9, 36–37. See also Obsessions

Educating others. See also Relationships
    building a support network and, 109
    dealing with negativity and, 111–112
    family relationships and, 129
    professional or educational environments
        and, 161
    questions from others, 90–91, 94, 159–160

requesting accommodations and, 159–160
    romantic relationships and, 148
    sharing your OCD story and, 86
Educating yourself, 161, 187, 198
Embarrassment, 108–110
Emotional distress. See also Fear; Guilt;
    Shame
    exposure and response prevention and, 17,
        180–181
    family relationships and, 116, 125
    overview, 8–11
    romantic relationships and, 131, 144
    sharing your OCD story and, 86
Emotional intelligence, 101
Emotions. See also Emotional distress
    celebrating success and resilience and,
        30–31
    crises and, 168–169, 178
    cycle of OCD and, 11–15, 15f
    responding to reactions from others and, 94
Empathy
    building a support network and, 100, 107
    professional or educational environments
        and, 161
    sharing your OCD story and, 93–94
    understanding of OCD and, 8
Empowerment, 96–97, 181
Enjoyable activities. See also Activities
    crises and, 172–173
    discovering your true self and, 25
    exposure and response prevention and,
        191–192
    family relationships and, 129
    identity beyond OCD and, 32–33, 35
    overcoming procrastination and, 80
    romantic relationships and, 141, 143, 148
    selecting rewards and, 32–33
Evidence for and against obsessions, 43–49
Exercise. See Physical activity
Expectations, 23, 169
Exposure and response prevention (ERP).
    See also Professional help
    adjusting when it seems ineffective,
        192–195
    myths and misunderstandings regarding,
        180–183
    optimizing the effects of, 5
    overview, 1–3, 4, 16–18, 36, 179–180,
        189–190, 196–197, 198
    reducing OCD symptoms and, 16–19
    roadblocks to, 184–188
    strategies for long-term success with,
        195–196
    strategies for overcoming roadblocks,
        186–192

Family relationships. *See also* Relationships
conflicts related to OCD and, 124–128
crises and, 167–168
exposure and response prevention and,
   185, 188, 189–190, 194, 198
family communication patterns, 118–124
getting support from family and friends
   and, 61–63
OCD within the family context and,
   115–118
overview, 5, 11, 115, 128, 129
problem solving and decision making and,
   122–124
sharing your OCD story and, 84–89
Fear. *See also* Emotional distress; Obsessions
building a support network and, 108–110
of change, 186
crises and, 164, 169–176
exposure and response prevention and,
   16–17, 18, 181, 184–186
negative reinforcement loop and, 15*f*
OCD within the family context and, 116,
   117
overview, 8, 9, 21, 36–37
reducing OCD symptoms and, 16
romantic relationships and, 131, 137–139
sharing your OCD story and, 107–108
Feared self, 44–45
Feedback, 30–31
Feelings, 168–169, 178. *See also* Emotional
   distress; Emotions
Flexibility, 76, 102–103, 144, 151, 163
Flooding, 170–171. *See also* Crisis
   management
Friendships, 11, 61–63. *See also* Relationships

Goals
compared to values, 27–28
crises and, 169
framing affirmations as, 26
moving towards core values and, 28–29
professional or educational environments
   and, 160
for resisting compulsive urges, 64
Growth, personal. *See* Personal growth
Guilt. *See also* Emotional distress
celebrating success and resilience and,
   29–31
core values and, 26–29, 27*f*
crises and, 173–174
discovering your true self and, 24–26
identity beyond OCD and, 31–33
overview, 2, 4, 21–22, 34

replacing with self-compassion, 35
romantic relationships and, 139

Habituation, 17, 181
Hand-washing rituals. *See* Washing behaviors
Harm-related obsessions, 9, 131
Health-related crises, 172–173. *See also* Crisis
   management
Helping others, 33, 35
Hobbies
crises and, 172–173
identity beyond OCD and, 32–33, 35
recovering from a breakup and, 147
selecting rewards from, 64
Household crises and accidents, 170–172. *See
   also* Crisis management

"I" statements. *See also* Communication
dealing with negativity and, 112–113
family communication patterns, 118–119,
   129
OCD-related family conflicts and, 127
sharing your OCD story and, 90
Identity, 24–26, 31–33, 34, 35
Impact of OCD
crises and, 165
discovering your true self and, 25
on the family, 115–118
romantic relationships and, 131–133,
   140–145
at work or in the classroom, 149–151
Important tasks. *See also* Prioritizing tasks
ABCD method strategy and, 72–74
Activity Log and, 71
overcoming procrastination and, 79–81
overview, 68–69
structuring days to minimize OCD's
   interference, 74–77
Individuals with Disabilities Education Act
   (IDEA), 155
Inference-based cognitive behavioral therapy
   (I-CBT), 36, 43–45
Inferential confusion, 42–45
Injury, 173. *See also* Crisis management
Intimacy, physical, 132, 133–136, 148. *See
   also* Romantic relationships
Intrusive thoughts. *See also* Obsessions;
   Symptoms; Thoughts
changing your perspective on obsessions
   and, 37–42
cycle of OCD and, 11–15, 15*f*
discrediting obsessions and, 42–49

negative reinforcement loop and, 13–14, 15*f*
overview, 9
romantic relationships and, 131, 134–135, 137–138
Isolation
cycle of, 105–107, 114
obstacles to seeking support and, 105–107
OCD-related family conflicts and, 125
sharing your OCD story and, 96–97
support from others and, 104

Job loss, 175. *See also* Crisis management; Workplace environment
Judgement, 100, 110–113, 122

Legal rights, 154–160
Leisure, 27–28, 27*f*, 64. *See also* Enjoyable activities
Limit setting, 111–112, 148. *See also* Boundaries

Mediation, 127–128
Medical diagnosis, 172–173. *See also* Crisis management
Medications, 1–2, 5, 16, 192
Mental rituals. *See also* Compulsions and compulsive rituals; Rituals
exposure and response prevention and, 18
modifying rituals and, 58
overview, 8, 10
romantic relationships and, 132
Mindfulness techniques, 153, 193–194, 198
Misinterpretations, 12–13, 15*f*, 16
Mistakes and guilt, 173–174. *See also* Crisis management; Guilt
Misunderstandings, 116–117, 125. *See also* Communication
Modifying rituals, 57–58, 137, 166

Negative reinforcement loop, 13–18, 15*f*
Negativity from others, 110–113
Nonverbal behavior, 120

Objectifying unwanted thoughts strategy, 40
Obsessions. *See also* Anxiety; Doubts; Fear; Symptoms; Thoughts; Uncertainty
Activity Log and, 71
changing your perspective on, 37–42, 50

crises and, 164, 168–176
cycle of OCD and, 11–15, 15*f*
delaying rituals and, 55–56
discrediting, 42–49, 50
explaining to others, 90–91, 92
exposure and response prevention and, 16–18, 181–183
negative reinforcement loop and, 13–14
OCD within the family context and, 116
overview, 2–3, 4, 8–11, 36–37
reducing OCD symptoms and, 16
romantic relationships and, 131, 137–139, 148
Obsessive compulsive disorder (OCD) overview
cycle of OCD and, 11–15, 15*f*
explaining to others, 90–91, 92
overview, 8–11, 18–19
OCD story, 44, 45–49. *See also* Sharing your OCD story with others
Online support groups, 104, 106. *See also* Support groups; Support networks
Organization, 11, 67, 77–78, 152–153, 163. *See also* Routines; Time management

Paper-and-pencil planner. *See* Planner use
Passions, 32–33, 35
Patience, 102–103, 169
Patterns, 8, 10, 54. *See also* Compulsions and compulsive rituals
Peer support, 103–105. *See also* Support networks
Perfectionism, 91, 135–136, 175–176
Personal growth. *See also* Self-acceptance; Self-compassion
academic crises and, 176
celebrating, 29–31
core values and, 27–28, 27*f*
overview, 23
understanding of OCD and, 8
Perspective on obsessions, 37–42, 43–49, 50, 166. *See also* Obsessions
Pest infestation, 171. *See also* Crisis management
Physical activity, 60, 153, 168, 173, 178
Planner use, 74–77, 152–153. *See also* Time management
Pomodoro technique, 78
Positive reinforcement, 63–65, 166
Possibility trap, 47–48
Practice in ERP, 183, 193, 198
Prioritizing tasks. *See also* Time management
Activity Log, 69–72, 70*f*
breaking down complex tasks, 75, 80–81

Prioritizing tasks (*continued*)
crises and, 178
important versus urgent tasks, 68–69
overcoming procrastination and, 79–81
overview, 68–74, 70f, 82
professional or educational environments and, 151–152, 163
Privacy. *See also* Sharing your OCD story with others
myths about sexuality and relationship dynamics and, 136
overview, 83–84, 86
romantic relationships and, 136, 139
social media and, 89
Problem solving
academic crises and, 176
active listening and, 122
family communication patterns and, 122–124
OCD-related family conflicts and, 126–128
overview, 10–11
Procrastination, 79–81, 82. *See also* Time management
Professional help. *See also* Exposure and response prevention (ERP); Treatment
building a support network and, 108, 109
continued treatment and, 196
crises and, 168–169
finding the right therapist, 188, 191
OCD-related family conflicts and, 128
overview, 15, 96
recovering from a breakup and, 147
romantic relationships and, 145
Pros and cons strategy, 85, 86, 98
Purpose, sense of, 33, 35

Questions from others, 90–91, 94, 159–160. *See also* Educating others; Sharing your OCD story with others

Reactions from others, 93–96, 98, 108. *See also* Sharing your OCD story with others
Reassurance from others, 142, 144, 185
Reassurance seeking, 10, 60, 148. *See also* Compulsions and compulsive rituals
Reciprocity, 101–102
Reflection, 78, 120–121, 151, 195–196
Relapse, 86, 196
Relationship OCD (ROCD), 131, 135–136, 138–139

Relationships. *See also* Educating others; Family relationships; Friendships; Romantic relationships; Sharing your OCD story with others; Support networks
building a support network and, 100–101, 114
core values and, 27–28, 27f
crises and, 167–168
cycle of isolation and, 106
dealing with negativity and, 110–113, 114
exposure and response prevention and, 185, 188, 189–190, 194, 198
overview, 4–5, 11
self-compassion and self-acceptance and, 23
sharing your OCD story and, 84–89, 98
unsupportive relationships and, 110–113, 114
Relaxation strategies, 33, 153, 173
Reminders, 73, 153
Resilience
celebrating, 29–31
charting, 29–30
overview, 4, 34, 35
rewarding, 31
self-compassion and self-acceptance and, 23
Responses from others, 93–96, 98, 108. *See also* Sharing your OCD story with others
Responsibility, 9, 117, 174
Rewards, 63–65, 80. *See also* Celebrating progress
Riding the waves of compulsive urges, 56–57, 64–65, 137
Ritual Awareness Log, 52–55, 53f, 66, 196
Ritual delay or modification, 55–58, 137, 166
Rituals. *See also* Compulsions and compulsive rituals; Mental rituals; Symptoms
awareness of, 52–55, 53f
competing responses and, 58–61, 66
delaying, 55–57, 66
exposure and response prevention and, 17, 18
modifying, 57–58, 66
negative reinforcement loop and, 13–14, 15f
OCD within the family context and, 116
overview, 2–3, 8, 10–11, 51, 65, 66
positive reinforcement and, 63–65
prioritizing tasks and, 69

reducing OCD symptoms and, 16
rewarding yourself for, 66
romantic relationships and, 131–132, 137–139, 140, 142
support from others and, 61–63, 66
Romantic relationships. *See also* Relationships
breakups and, 146–147
effects of OCD on, 131–133
managing OCD symptoms in, 137–139
myths about sexuality and relationship dynamics and, 133–136
overview, 5, 11, 130, 148
reducing accommodations within, 141–145
resolving conflicts and, 145–146
sharing your OCD story and, 87–88
working with your partner to manage OCD, 140–145
Routines. *See also* Schedules; Time management
ABCD method strategy and, 72–74
conflicts related to OCD and, 125
crises and, 167, 171–172, 178
exposure and response prevention and, 18, 198
family relationships and, 116, 125
incorporating affirmations into, 25–26
modifying rituals and, 57–58
professional or educational environments and, 151, 163
recovering from a breakup and, 146–147
romantic relationships and, 142
social interactions and, 107
structuring days to minimize OCD's interference, 74–77, 82

Schedules. *See also* Activities; Calendar use; Planner use; Routines; Time management
crises and, 178
professional or educational environments and, 151, 163
recovering from a breakup and, 146–147
romantic relationships and, 148
structuring days to minimize OCD's interference, 74–77
School functioning
core values and, 27–28, 27f
crisis management, 175–176
dealing with negativity from teachers and, 112–113
effects of OCD on, 149–151

legal rights to accommodations and, 154–160
long-term strategies for success and, 160–162
overview, 5, 11, 149, 163
requesting accommodations and, 158, 159–160
strategies for managing OCD at school and, 151–154
Section 504 of the Rehabilitation Act of 1973, 155
Security concerns, 170. *See also* Crisis management
Selective serotonin reuptake inhibitors (SSRIs), 1–2, 5, 16. *See also* Medications
Self-acceptance
celebrating, 29–31
core values and, 26–29, 27f
discovering your true self and, 24–26
fostering, 24–26
identity beyond OCD and, 31–33
overview, 4, 22–23, 34, 35
sharing your OCD story and, 86, 96–97
Self-advocacy, 176
Self-care, 76, 146–147, 168, 178
Self-compassion. *See also* Personal growth
ABCD method strategy and, 74
building a support network and, 108, 109
celebrating, 29–31
crises and, 169, 174, 178
making mistakes and, 174
overview, 22–23, 34, 35
professional or educational environments and, 153–154
Self-concept, 24–26
Self-directed ERP, 195. *See also* Exposure and response prevention (ERP)
Self-esteem, 18, 63
Self-stigma, 4, 11, 19, 24. *See also* Stigma
Sex, unwanted thoughts of, 9, 131, 134–135
Sexual functioning, 5, 132, 133–136. *See also* Romantic relationships
Sexual orientation, 135
Shame. *See also* Emotional distress
building a support network and, 108–110
celebrating success and resilience and, 29–31
core values and, 26–29, 27f
discovering your true self and, 24–26
identity beyond OCD and, 31–33
overview, 2, 4, 9, 11, 19, 21–22, 34
replacing with self-compassion, 35
sharing your OCD story and, 96–97

Sharing your OCD story with others. *See also* Relationships
  building a support network and, 96–97, 107–108, 114
  communication strategies for, 90–93
  considerations in, 84–89
  expanding the circle of people you share with, 107–108
  fear regarding, 107–108, 114
  obstacles to seeking support and, 107–108
  overview, 83–84, 97, 98
  questions from others, 90–91, 94, 159–160
  requesting workplace accommodations, 156
  responding to reactions to, 93–96, 98, 108
  romantic relationships and, 130, 136, 139
  sample scripts for, 92–93
  seeking help and support and, 96–97
Sleep, 168, 178
Smartphones, 153. *See also* Technology use; Tools
Social activities, 106–107, 117, 125. *See also* Activities
Social boundaries. *See* Boundaries
Social functioning, 18, 125
Social media, 32–33, 89
Social relationships. *See* Relationships
Social support. *See* Support networks
Stigma
  building a support network and, 108–110
  obstacles to seeking support and, 105
  self-stigma, 4, 11, 19, 24
  sharing your OCD story and, 86, 94
Strengths, 29–33, 34, 176
Stress
  crises and, 177
  cycle of isolation and, 105
  family relationships and, 116, 125
  professional or educational environments and, 153–154
Structure, 74–77, 82, 151. *See also* Organization; Routines; Time management
Support groups. *See also* Support networks
  cycle of isolation and, 106
  exposure and response prevention and, 188
  overview, 103–104
  recovering from a breakup and, 147
  romantic relationships and, 145
Support networks. *See also* Relationships; Support groups
  crises and, 167–168, 171, 172–174
  cycle of isolation and, 105–107
  dealing with negativity and, 110–113

  enhancing, 100–103
  exposure and response prevention and, 188, 189–190, 194, 198
  obstacles to seeking support, 105–113
  overview, 4–5, 99, 114
  recovering from a breakup and, 147
  rituals and, 61–63
  seeking positive feedback from, 30–31
  sharing your OCD story and, 86, 96–97
  specialized support and, 103–105
  understanding of OCD and, 8
Surfing the compulsive urges, 56–57, 64–65, 137
Symptoms. *See also* Avoidance; Compulsions and compulsive rituals; Obsessions; Rituals
  crises and, 165–169, 178
  cycle of isolation and, 105
  dealing with negativity and, 111–112
  explaining to others, 90–91
  exposure and response prevention and, 185
  OCD within the family context and, 115–118
  overview, 4, 8–11
  procrastination and, 79
  professional or educational environments and, 160–162
  reducing, 15–19
  romantic relationships and, 137–139, 148

Tasks. *See* Breaking down tasks; Prioritizing tasks
Teachers, 112–113
Technology use. *See also* Tools
  online support groups and, 104, 106
  professional or educational environments and, 153
  sharing your OCD story and, 89
  time management and, 77
Therapists, finding the right one, 188, 191. *See also* Exposure and response prevention (ERP); Professional help
Thoughts. *See also* Intrusive thoughts; Obsessions
  changing your perspective on obsessions and, 37–42
  crises and, 168–169, 178
  cycle of OCD and, 11–15, 15*f*
  discrediting obsessions and, 42–49
  exposure and response prevention and, 17
  negative reinforcement loop and, 13–14
  overview, 8, 36–37
  romantic relationships and, 137–138

Time management. *See also* Activities;
     Organization; Routines; Schedules
  ABCD method strategy, 72–74
  Activity Log, 69–72
  minimizing distractions, 77–78
  overcoming procrastination, 79–81
  overview, 11, 67–68, 81, 82
  prioritizing tasks, 68–74, 70*f*
  professional or educational environments
     and, 151–152
  structuring days to minimize OCD's
     interference and, 74–77
Time with supporters, 102. *See also* Support
     networks
Timers, 76–77
To-do lists, 152–153
Tools, 73, 74–77, 89, 152–153. *See also*
     Technology use
Transforming obsessions into an object
     strategy, 40
Treatment, 1–3, 15–19, 91, 198. *See also*
     Exposure and response prevention
     (ERP); Professional help
Triggers
  crises and, 165, 169
  explaining to others, 91
  exposure and response prevention and,
     181
  family relationships and, 117, 124–126
  negative reinforcement loop and, 15*f*
  perception flip strategy and, 46–47
  procrastination and, 79
  Ritual Awareness Log and, 52–55, 53*f*
Trust, 87, 101, 107

Uncertainty, 8, 9. *See also* Obsessions
Understanding, 86, 107
Understanding Exposure and Response
     Prevention (ERP) for OCD handout,
     188, 189–190

Unsupportive relationships, 110–113, 114. *See
     also* Relationships
Urgent tasks. *See also* Prioritizing tasks
  ABCD method strategy and, 72–74
  Activity Log and, 71
  overview, 68–69
  structuring days to minimize OCD's
     interference, 74–77
Using distraction strategy, 60–61

Validation from others, 96–97
Values, core. *See* Core values
Values Target exercise, 27–29, 27*f*
Volunteer work, 33, 35

Washing behaviors, 10, 59, 131–132. *See
     also* Compulsions and compulsive rituals
Wasting time, 71–72. *See also* Time
     management
Water leakage, 170–171. *See also* Crisis
     management
Workplace environment
  core values and, 27–28, 27*f*
  crisis management, 175
  dealing with negativity from bosses and,
     112–113
  effects of OCD on, 149–151
  exposure and response prevention and, 18
  job loss and, 175
  legal rights to accommodations and, 154–160
  long-term strategies for success and,
     160–162
  overview, 11, 149, 163
  requesting accommodations and, 156–158,
     159–160
  sharing your OCD story and, 86, 88
  strategies for managing OCD at work and,
     151–154
  workspace and, 77–78

about the author

Jonathan S. Abramowitz, PhD, ABPP, is Professor of Psychology and Neuroscience and Research Professor of Psychiatry at the University of North Carolina (UNC) at Chapel Hill. He is also Director of the UNC Clinical Psychology PhD Training Program. Dr. Abramowitz conducts research on OCD and other anxiety-related disorders and has published over 20 books and 300 peer-reviewed research articles and book chapters. He is Founding Editor in Chief of the *Journal of Obsessive–Compulsive and Related Disorders* and serves on the editorial boards of several other scientific journals. Dr. Abramowitz is a scientific and clinical advisory board member for the International OCD Foundation and a past president of the Association for Behavioral and Cognitive Therapies. He has received numerous awards for his contributions to the fields of OCD and clinical psychology and for his mentorship of students and trainees. His books include *The Family Guide to Getting Over OCD*, *Getting Over OCD, Second Edition*, and *The Stress Less Workbook* (for general readers), and *Exposure Therapy for Anxiety, Second Edition* (for mental health professionals).